Becoming
Naturally
You

Becoming Naturally You

39 Simple Steps To Naturally Transform Your Mind, Diet & Life

Leah Salmon

Naturally You Presents

Leah Salmon's

Becoming Naturally You

39 Simple Steps To Naturally Transform Your Health & Life

Published 2009
Revised 2013
Revised 2015

© Leah Salmon 2015

ISBN: 978-0-9926422-9-7

Whilst every effort has been made to ensure that the information contained in this book is accurate and up to date, it is advisory only and should not be used as an alternative to seeking qualified professional advice. The author and publisher cannot be held responsible for actions or omissions that may be taken by the reader as a result of reliance on the information contained in this book. The information is taken entirely at the reader's own risk.

This book is dedicated to

My Beautiful Mother Jennifer David
*Possibly the kindest, strongest and most beautiful woman
I've had the pleasure of knowing, Love you mummy*

My Father and Teacher Paa Nabab Yaanun
*This powerful being is more than my teacher, more than my
father, more than my guide, he has saved my life and
inspired my work on so many occasions and for this I will
love and respect him always*

Amun Sekhemu Ankh Shimsuwn Elijah Salmon
My little guardian angel

**Shaep, Mattat, Sakhamtat, Anqat, Khafrayay, Nafurtat &
Nuntat Salmon**
My best friend and beautiful ones

Julian Hall The Ultrapreneur
*The "you can do it" behind every doubt I have in myself,
tawuhtak*

*A special thank you also goes out to all my family, friends,
ancestors and descendants.*

Contents

Introducing Becoming Naturally You

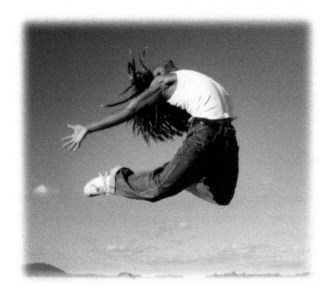

According to modern science…

It takes just over 39 weeks for a baby to fully form in the womb of its mother. That's pretty quick considering a brand new human, made from scratch comes out. Now, imagine in the next 39 weeks you could transform your mind, diet and body, to feel brand new, would you do it?

Well if you think you're up to it, this book is a great place to start.

This is a slightly revised version of my very first book "The Ultimate You" and just like it's predecessor, this book is a 39 step guide to making simple weekly changes, that can individually have a positive effect on your short term health and cumulatively transform the way you eat, think and live.

Having had a few children myself, well 6 to be exact, I know the 39-40 weeks of pregnancy can fly by, when every week brings a new change or challenge, and especially if you use one of those pregnancy apps or calendars with the week by week development of your baby. Babies go through huge changes and developments each week, even if on the surface, you only get a pound or two bigger and an inch wider.

The same could be true for you.

By committing to small regular changes each week, you can undergo a slow, steady and powerful development, that doesn't seem overwhelming, unmanageable or too fast for you to keep up with.

Is Our Diet The Only Important Thing In Life?

A few years ago I realised that helping people improve their diet, by removing processed nutrient robbing junk foods and replacing them with nutrient dense whole foods could be tremendously beneficial to their lives and I loved seeing the results of the work I did with people. But it also became apparent that it was one piece of a very important puzzle called LIFE.

My focus was on ensuring my clients were nourished and fulfilled nutritionally, but what about their career, their family life, their relationships, their life goals and aspirations. What could they do to be nourished in those areas too?

Your food is your fuel so it's paramount that you get that right so you have the energy to work on the other areas of your life. But I realised how important it was that I also helped people to work on the other areas of their life so they would create balance in their development, instead of getting really great results in their health, while they did nothing to get out of a job they hate and a relationship that was suffocating them, for example.

I've also learned from bitter experience that when you only focus on one area of your life and not others, the negative energy from any difficult areas can make it hard for you to remain focused on developing any areas.

It's like when you put off dealing with your health while you fully focus on your career, and as your career success reaches a peak, your health has been sufficiently ignored to the point where it literally stops you in your tracks, meaning you can't enjoy the results of the career success you've attained or worse still, all the career success you've gained is now lost as you struggle to regain your health.

Balance is key

So I created a new way of working with people, which focused on helping people to create a LIFE **that nourished and fulfilled them on every level**, mainly through getting rid of negative beliefs that hold us back and creating workable plans that get us to our health and life goals as quickly as possible.

So this book has been revised with this goal in mind, to help you create a life that nourishes and fulfils you on every level, with small weekly manageable steps that transform your diet, body and mind naturally in under 10 months.

How To Use The Book

The book Is laid out in step by step format, so you can easily work your way through it one step a week. The steps are sectioned into 3 main areas, which are:

1) Mind & Environment Steps – We're going to start by getting your thoughts and environment in a state where they can positively support all the changes you'll be making with your foods and body. Not having the right mindset to begin with can be the downfall of many worthy endeavours.

2) Foods Steps – This is where we look specifically at the actual foods and drinks you put into your body and how you can make them as wholesome as possible.

3) Body Steps – This is where we look at things you can do to physically improve your body, from exercise and breathing to cleansing and sleeping.

You simply read the pages for a step, work on that step for a week, use the journaling pages and tips to track your progress, then move onto reading the section for the next week, complete that week and keep going.

There's a "Cover To Cover" checklist of the steps at the back of the book so you can see how far you've gotten and how far you have to go.

If you want to speed things up and work on 2 steps a week, use the "Fast Track Plan" at the back and finish in half the time, ready to continue your life long journey.

If you're the type of person who prefers to read the whole book first (like me) then decide what steps you want to take and in what order, there's a "My 39 Steps Plan" at the back of the book you can use to fill in your own order of following the steps and keep track on them.

Fancy a more exciting life?!? Use "The Variety Plan" at the back, which mixes the steps up from the 3 sections.

However you decide to use this book, I hope very soon you begin to feel the benefits of becoming nourished and fulfilled on every level, as a result of Becoming Naturally You.

"One small change a week, will speed up the change you seek"

Leah Salmon

What Does Becoming Naturally You Mean To You

Before we get started, take a moment to think about what Becoming Naturally You means to you. What does being nourished and fulfilled on every level actually look like for you? Fill in the questions below, continue on more paper if needed so you can have a clear vision in your mind of how you want your life to turn out.

This is what my life would look like if I was being Naturally Me and felt nourished and fulfilled on every level:

My nourishing and fulfilling environment would include

_____

_____

_____

_____

It wouldn't include: -

_____Excessive biscuits, sweet_____

_____Cakes_____

My nourished and fulfilled mind would be full of thoughts of

_____

_____

_____

_____

Becoming Naturally You

It wouldn't have thoughts of

Take-aways

My nourishing and fulfilling diet would be full of yummy

fruit e vegetables

It wouldn't include:

Chocolate sweets
crisps biscuits -

My nourished and fulfilled body would (look/feel/have)

less stomach felt.

It wouldn't (look/feel/have):

flabby

To me, Becoming Naturally Me means:

_____

_____

_____

_____

_____

_____

3 of the reasons it's important for me to Become Naturally Me are

1. _____

_____

_____

2. _____

_____

_____

3. _____

_____

_____

Your Becoming Naturally You Mind & Environment Steps

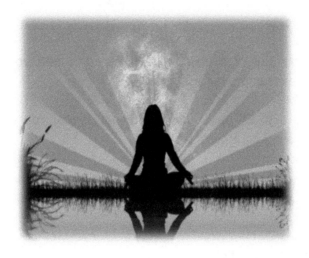

"All that you achieve and all that you fail to achieve, is a direct result of your own thoughts"

That pretty much sums up this section.

Before you venture into anything, your mind has to see the positive end results first, or at the very least accept the fact that positive results are a definite possibility.

On the first day of a new class, you need to see yourself holding a pass certificate.

On the first day of a new job, you need to see yourself being promoted over and over again.

When you sign up for your first driving lesson, you need to see yourself driving your own car.

Before you even start writing a business plan to start your own business, you need to see yourself successfully established in business.

As an athlete or artist; train, practice and perform like you have already won gold or a Grammy.

It all starts in your head.

Being in a supportive and nurturing environment can do wonders for your rate of success. So even though some will succeed no matter where they are, prevention is better than cure. Let's not let a toxic mind or environment sabotage the success you can achieve during this process. Discover the simple steps you can take to control your mind and environment to encourage your success by working through this first set of steps.

Here's to your success!

Step 1 – Potential Trouble Sources

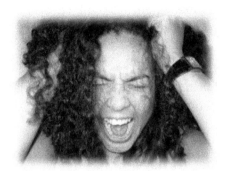 Everyone has their pet hates, mild irritations and things that rub them up the wrong way. We can pretty much live with these things without them getting in the way of our progress.

But there are some things or people that can literally ruin our day by just being there, completely bring us down in a way that makes it difficult to get up again, these are potential trouble sources or PTSs.

As you embark upon this journey to Becoming Naturally You, you're likely to experience ups and downs, moments where you're joyfully blissful and others where you doubt having ever started. During this time, the last thing you need is for anyone or anything to encourage the negative thoughts that could crop up, which are very often little lies our subconscious feeds us to keep us from experiencing change, the type of change that is necessary for growth.

The definition of a **Potential Trouble Source** or **PTS** is something or someone that sets you off into a negative state of mind. You might call them or it an "energy sucker" or just simply very negative. Unless you are of a certain mind set, where you always expect greatness for yourself, have a really positive mental attitude and are very focused on your personal goals for self improvement, which unfortunately very few people are, you MUST disassociate yourself with all PTSs NOW!!!

These are the things you will normally hear from a PTS or suppressive person as they are also known:

"You'll never lose that much weight"

"What's the point in doing that, it won't work"

"That's a lot of money to spend on yourself when you've got so many debts"

"You'll never afford that"

"Don't waste your time trying that, it'll never work"

"Haven't you tried every diet already, what makes this one so special"

"You should just be happy with the little you have"

"Your expectations are a bit high aren't they" - Sound familiar...

There are two ways to deal with these types of people, you could avoid them at all costs, but if that's not possible, you need to find a way of dealing with them. A friend of mine says that her aunt is her PTS and whenever she starts being negative, she'll imagine her with tweetie birds flying around her head chirping. It works a treat apparently!

There are also things that can act as PTSs, such as

The News – 80% of the news is sharing tragedy and disaster, none of which is going to keep your energy high and positive. If you want to keep up to date with the latest world news, set aside a small amount of time for this once a week, limit it as much as possible, even if just for the length of this process.

Social Media – It obviously depends on who you follow and what you do on social media, but just like the news, you can never be sure exactly what you'll be exposed to if you just sit and scroll though what everyone of your friends and their friends are posting. Use it for a purpose, don't be afraid to unfriend or unfollow and proceed with caution during this time!!!

Gossip websites, Gossip Magazines and Television – Just like the news, there's a heavy emphasis on scandalous stories sharing negative news about people you don't even know, none of which are going to positively motivate you to succeed in your health and life goals for the day.

At least 9 out of 10 of the most successful people I know in various fields and professions share this same opinion – TV, gossip columns and the news are a tiny part of their life, as they are a distraction that they have less and less time for, the more successful they become in their life.

Step 1 – Identify any PTSs you have in your life, work out whether you can avoid them and if not work out a way to best deal with them

It's likely that you'll only have one or two really influential PTSs that you need to deal with, so don't feel you need to break off all friendships, bin your TV and cut off your internet.

Identify any associations you need to break, even if temporarily and be fearless in doing it.

Often the best thing needed for growth is space

To make this step a success, this week I am committed to:

_____

_____

_____

_____

_____

_____

_____

_____

_____

_____

_____

By the end of this week I hope to:

_____

_____

_____

_____

_____

Step 2 – Write From The Heart

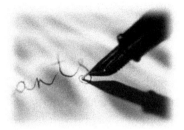

I always thought that journaling was something that hormonal teenage girls did in their bedroom after school.

I imagine pages of love hearts with their latest crush's name in them and reams of complaints about how unfair life is and how much they hate their parents. Back in my teenage years, a diary and the latest copy of Just Seventeen were always under my pillow, helping me find solace in the cruel world (I was soooooo dramatic as a teenager, blasted hormones).

The world has moved on a bit and now most teens (and adult) are on some form of social network sharing their every thought in anything from a 140 character tweet to a 20mins YouTube rant.

My use of a journal has changed somewhat since I was a teenager too and while there's no right or wrong way of journaling, here's a way I recommend and some of the benefits you can gain by doing it whilst you change your life and health for the better. You'll need:

The Journal

This is the notebook, diary or sheets of paper that you'll be using to write on, if you really prefer doing it digitally, then a word or text doc is sufficient, but there a different energy when you actually put pen to paper. These day's, we spend quite a lot of time in front of some form of screen so this can also serve as a break from gadgets for a moment. I decided to buy a really pretty wire bound notebook with glittery dolphins on the covers. I wanted something that looked pretty and special so that I'd enjoy picking it up and writing in it. If you aren't bothered with this then the next thing you need is...

The Pen
If you're going digital then this part won't apply to you, but I bought a fountain pen, nothing very expensive, but I do like writing with them so it matched the book in that respect. I kept them together and only used them together.

The Time
I have young children whose schedule and sleep patterns are constantly changing so it was tricky finding one set time to journal, but what I did do is make sure that there was at least 10 minutes in the day I'd find to do it. Try and fit it in on the way to or from work on the bus or train, in the bath at night, before you sleep, when you wake up, during your lunch break, while you're waiting for a kettle to boil, during the ad break of a TV program or whenever you can.

What to do
Just listen and write. Sit for a moment, listen to yourself and write whatever comes to you. You could ask yourself a question like:

How are you feeling today?
How was work?
Exactly what did your husband/wife do to upset you?
Was it really necessary to shout at the children like that?
Was my best friend really being thoughtless with the comment they made or was I just feeling sensitive?
Wasn't it amazing how well the day went today?
Wasn't it lovely how my relative called to check up on me, what can I do for them?

Then simply answer the questions. Or you could just write an account of your day and what's happened since the last time you wrote.

It's like a running commentary of your life and thoughts put down on paper for you to read back to yourself. You could also use it to make sure you stick to your goals and if you slip up, you can write what happened. You could also use it to simply list your accomplishments for that day and what you want to accomplish the next day. How much you write is entirely up to you.

Why Journal?
This is a thoroughly cleansing, thought provoking, problems solving, soul growing, voyage of discovery to go on daily or as often as you can. When you go through changes in life, ups and downs, more often than not, you'll talk to everyone but yourself about it, when we should discuss it with ourselves first.

If you let your writing just flow, all the questions in your head will come out onto that paper, all your fears, hopes, dreams, goals and plans. Finally, you'll have them out of your head, making it so much easier to actually work on them.

It can be a form of therapy and many therapists actually recommend it to their clients as you get to confidentially express issues you have with yourself and others that could be stopping your progress in many areas of your life. You may find, as I have, that it's like the best friend you never had, and other times just a good read on a quiet day.

Step 29 – Journal your week for a full 7 days, starting from Sunday night to Saturday morning for example, and on Saturday evening read the whole thing back to yourself. See if you can make a little more sense out of your life by the end of it

If you write 10 words on the first day that's fine

If you fill 25 pages on the first day (yes I know people who have done that) that's fine

If want to journal in doodles and pictures, or song lyrics and poetry, that's fine

What's most important is that you start the process of cleansing and progression through writing and journaling and enjoy the journey and 'me time' that comes with it.

To make this step a success, this week I am committed to:

_____

_____

_____

_____

_____

_____

_____

_____

_____

_____

_____

By the end of this week I hope to:

_____

_____

_____

_____

_____

Step 3 – Stress Busting

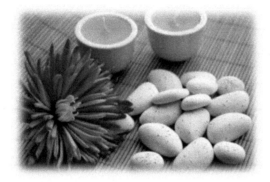 I used to work in a hospital, as a medical secretary first then as a nurse for a few years. It was a very interesting place to work.

While working as a secretary, which could be quite busy at times, my boss, a wonderful woman who was very good at her job, would always smile and say 'Leah, I'm too blessed to be stressed'. I loved hearing those words, it would always perk me up.

Something as simple as a positive thought was just what I needed to put my stress into perspective and transform it's energy into motivation to keep going.

You've probably heard the expression that 'Stress is a Killer', well on many levels this is very true.

The definition of stress is difficult for many medical and mental health experts to agree on, as it comes in so many forms with varying degrees of severity, but according to one dictionary it's defined as:

1. A specific response by the body to a stimulus, as fear or pain, that disturbs or interferes with the normal physiological equilibrium of an organism

28

2. Physical, mental, or emotional strain or tension: *Worry over his job and his wife's health put him under a great stress*
3. A situation, occurrence, or factor causing this: *The stress of being trapped in the elevator gave him a pounding headache*

Whenever the body is out of balance or equilibrium in any way, there is the potential of disease or illness to arise, on a mental, spiritual or physical level. So it's very important to have ways to deal with stress and stressful situations to keep yourself in balance as much as possible.

Stress manifests itself in many ways and some will be unique to the individual. One person could get a tension headache when they're stressed whilst someone else gets a rash on their arm, so we won't go into the symptoms of stress, but rather list a few ways you can deal with it.

• **Deep breathing** – Stress and tension can literally turn you into a rigid breathless knot. Your breathing will become extremely shallow, your shoulders go up and your head often drops down and forward, all of which you may not even notice until it's pointed out to you. When you feel yourself getting stressed, find a quite place (a bathroom, an empty room, the corridor, step outside for a moment) and take a few deep breaths (see Step 34).

This can help relieve stress by bringing oxygen into the brain and muscles that can energise them, making thinking clearer. Also taking a deep breath allows your shoulders to drop down from your ears relaxing them. It also temporarily distracts you from the source of stress, brings your focus back to nourishing your body and the situation may not seem so stressful once you've finished thie exercises.

- **Aromatherapy** – The best essential oils for combating stress are:

Lavender
Chamomile
Geranium
Clary Sage &
Sandalwood

I personally find Cedarwood and Jasmine oil really relaxing at stressful times, but I think that might just be because I love their rich, deep aroma.

This is an important point regarding aromatherapy, different oils have particular properties that can in many ways be proven (tea tree kills bacteria, peppermint perks you up, chamomile is very calming), however, as long as you exercise caution while using them, finding the one that resonates with you (which can be just that you really like its scent) and having it around when you need a pick me up, can work wonders too. You can simply open the bottle and have a sniff.

Inhaling them is often enough, but if you want to put them on your skin or both, it's safest to dilute them in a carrier oil first and check you aren't sensitive to it first.

- **Talking** – having someone to talk to about a situation that is causing you stress can be the best medicine. Talking to the right person can help you discover a way to deal with the situation so it no longer causes you stress. Journaling can also achieve this as the answers we seek are often already inside us.

- **Herbal Medicine** - Herbs can be drank as an infusion (tea) or added to a hot bath to act as mild and natural stress relievers. You could try:

Chamomile
Lemon balm
St John's Wort &
Valerian

You can also get these herbs in tinctures or herbal extracts, which are a bit easier to take with a higher potency. I'd advise you find the ones that don't contain alcohol so your body doesn't have to deal with this as well.

- **Water & Foods** – Stress can be made worse if you haven't eaten properly, haven't eaten the right foods or if you're dehydrated.

So make sure that during times and situations of stress, you keep well hydrated (drink at least 1 ½ litres of water throughout the day, see Step 13), eat right for your metabolic type so you get the most energy from your food (see step 23) and avoid things that negatively affect your blood sugar levels and mental function in general, like high levels of refined sugar, foods heavily fried in low quality oils, alcohol, narcotics and processed junk foods.

- **Stretch those vocal cords** - After a long stressful day at work, put on the radio in your car and at the top of your voice, in 6pm traffic, sing any of the following for instant stress relief (well it'll put a smile on someone's face):

Pointer Sisters	Jump For My Love
Diane Ross	Chain Reaction
Bob Marley	Don't Worry About A Thing
Aerosmith	Don't Want To Miss A Thing
Smash Mouth	Hey Now You're An All Star
Bee Gees	Staying Alive
Village People	YMCA
Bob Marley	One Love
Pharrelle Williams	Happy
Jimmy Cliff	I Can See Clearly Now
Aretha Franklin	Respect

- **Move about** – Whether you go for a run, lift some weights or put some music on and dance, even if it's the last thing you feel like doing, again it can lift your mood, distract you and get the oxygen flowing.

- **Cuddles** – Having someone to give you a great big bear hug is a lovely way to improve your mood. Apparently...

> Cuddling literally kills depression, relieves anxiety and strengthens the immune system.

- **Self Massage** – Most people go straight for their temples and give them a good rub in times of stress, whether there is pain there or not, it's just a relaxing instinct. You don't need to get out a massage table and towels at work to give yourself a quick stress busting massage. Try these simple techniques while sitting at your desk if you're at work, or just sitting somewhere comfy.

Self Massage Tips:

Head
Starting from the middle of your head, use both hands to rub all the way around your hairline in small, slow, steady circles as hard or soft as is most relaxing to you

Temples
Rub in small circles with your fingers

Neck
Rub down the center of your neck from your hairline to the top of your back

Shoulders
Rub and squeeze your shoulders from your neck to the corner of your shoulder and back again a few times. Circle your shoulders few times in between

Feet
Kick off your shoes under your desk and with your thumbs, massage as much of your foot as you can. Rotate your foot at the ankle and stretch it backwards and forwards.

Hands
Using the thumb on the opposite hand, massage as much of your hand as you can, rotate it at the wrist and stretch it backwards and forwards.

If you have a small bottle or tub of oil to use while doing this, all the better, but without is fine too.

Step 3 – **Choose any 3 of these stress busting methods to use daily over 7 days**

To make this step a success, this week I am committed to:

_____

_____

_____

_____

_____

_____

_____

_____

_____

By the end of this week I hope to:

_____

_____

_____

_____

Step 4 – Healthy Home Makeover

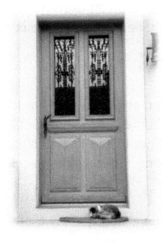

The environment in your home should be as nourishing, supportive and health giving as possible.

Clutter, mess, dirt, disorganisation can all stifle the productive energy in your home. So now's the time to give your home a healthy makeover.

This doesn't have to cost you a penny, simply moving things around, tidying up and doing some good old fashioned cleaning can do wonders for your home environment.

Here are some simple things you can change in your home to make it naturally more conducive to health.

Doorway
It's most important to keep your doorway tidy and uncluttered. Having to push the mess from around your doorway before you enter or leave your home is probably a reflection of congestion in other areas of your life too. Your door should be able to freely swing open and closed, for safety reasons if nothing else.

Place something near your doorway that can be seen as soon as you walk in, that really welcomes you; fresh flowers, pungent potpourri, a beautiful painting, a happy photograph or an ornament. If it's not possible, then hanging something beautiful

35

and decorative on your door doesn't just have to be reserved to a Christmas wreath or birthday balloons, it can be a permanent fixture to bring a smile to your face, that you can even periodically change as the mood takes you. Let it reflect who you are or what your family represents.

Kitchen

The kitchen is the heart of many homes and it's where the food is so it can make or break a healthy home. Food and family are inseparable, kitchens are meeting points in the home, places of comfort, socialising and of course eating. Four simple things you can do here are

1) Make sure junk foods are out of sight and healthy foods and snacks are readily available, so we're talking big fruit bowls and jugs of fresh water on the counter, and bags of crisps, cookie jars, cake stands (with cake on them) and soda at the back of the cupboard.

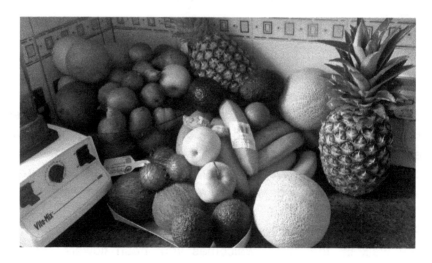

2) Keep your food and utensils well organised so when you want to prepare food, everything is easy to find and use. Don't keep the juicer packed away in the cupboard if you plan to make fresh juices 5 days a week.

In our kitchen, my 3 fruit bowls are out on the counter in between my food processor and juicer, the big bowls are in the cupboard below and the glasses are in the cupboard above. When I want a juice or a smoothie, I take a big bowl out, put the fruit I want to use in the bowl, then go to the fridge, add more produce to the bowl, wash them in the sink, come back to the counter, make the juice and pour it into the glasses in the cupboard above.

I also keep all my nuts, seeds and superfoods in one cupboard too so all the ingredients I need for protein shakes and raw nut sweets are together. My kitchen isn't massive so everything is no more than 10 steps away, if you have a bigger kitchen with things more spread out, consider moving things around to keep what you need for particular activities closer together.

3) Put up images of fresh healthy foods on the walls, I mean really delicious looking pictures that look good enough to eat, so that those are the things you want to eat when you go in there. Happy looking people eating those foods are helpful too.

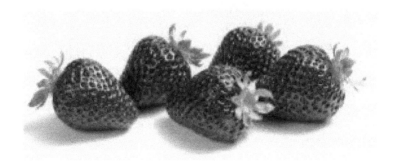

4) As with every room in the house, keeping it clean and tidy makes it more inviting, especially if you see food preparation as a chore. One of the best things you can do to improve your diet and chances of staying healthy, is to prepare as much of your own food as you can.

I know there are days when I go into my kitchen and if the dishes aren't done, I really don't want to prepare food until they are. This is when thoughts of getting take away or processed food creep in on me, but prevention is better than cure and this stage is about preventing anything that can delay or stop the success you can have when we get to the food steps.

Bathroom – Keeping your bathroom and toilet clean and sweet smelling is obviously a good move (though with a potty training baby girl and her absent minded siblings that can be a full time job in this house!!!) You can also jump forward to Step 36 and replace as many unnatural skincare and personal hygiene products as you can in your bathroom to keep the chemical fumes and residues away too.

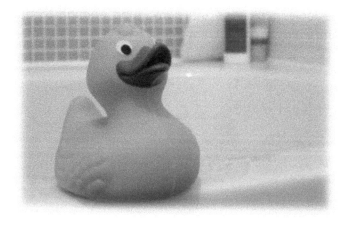

Bathroom & Kitchen Cleaning – Here are some natural cleaners you can use in your bathroom and kitchen instead of the harsher ones with harmful chemical bases.

Cleaner	Uses
Vinegar	Dilute 200mls with 200mls of water to de-scale your kettle and to wash fruit and vegetable skins to help remove some of the chemical residue. Use neat to wipe down counters, wash floors, clean windows and mirrors.
Lemon Juice	Add 6 used lemon peels to a mop bucket with hot water, let it sit for a while, then use the water to mop your floors.
Baking Soda (Bicarbonate of soda)	Add a little water to make a paste and place it on taps to remove lime scale. It can be added to your laundry wash to soften clothes and help remove stains and whiten clothes.
Borax	This naturally occurring substance is a great alternative to laundry powder without all the chemicals. Combine ½ a cup of borax with ½ cup of baking soda and a few drops of essential oil for scent, to wash a full load in your washing machine.
Tea Tree or Lemon Essential Oil	Add about 10 drops to a 5 litre mop bucket or about 5 drops to laundry powder to help kill harmful bacteria in your wash. Add to other cleaning fluids to naturally increase their antibacterial action.

"Chemical cleaners can leave poisons within us"

Leah Salmon

Living room – This is another room where family will congregate and get together to be social, so try and implement a TV time restriction in there. When the TV is on all the time, you lose precious bonding time with your family. Put on some background music and strike up a conversation, get some playing cards or a board game out or encourage your children to spend some time reading, writing or even dancing.

Office / Study – If you don't have a separate office, then wherever you normally have your computer or laptop, which are in most homes these days, get some crystals and gemstones like clear quartz, fluorite or Himalayan salt crystals and place them near your monitor or laptop to absorb the radiation that they emit.

If you have a desk that you sit at, use a Swiss ball instead of a chair the whole time and take breaks to prevent you from sitting down for prolonged periods of time, and make sure the room is well ventilated. When we're engrossed in computer based work, surfing the internet, watching TV or even reading, we can stop breathing properly (refer to Step 34) so a good supply of oxygen is helpful. You might have just caught yourself shallow breathing now that I've mentioned it!!!

This would be a good place to put inspirational posters and your vision board, which I talk more about in Step 10.

Bedrooms – The 7 best things you can do to make your bedroom as health promoting as possible are:

1) Keep it dust free: You sleep in here so if it's full of dust, you'll be breathing it in all night, which could eventually irritate your respiratory system.

2) Keep it well ventilated: A fresh air supply while you sleep is good for health. If you can safely do so, open your window a little while you sleep or just before go to bed to air the room out.

3) Try to only use this room for sleep and relaxing activities: Working, study and especially having the dreaded TV in your bedroom all change the energy in the room to make it more stimulating, which isn't conducive to restful sleep. Unless you are pushed for space, avoid this.

4) Keep it pitch black at night – this helps you get a more rested sleep. If you can't block out all the lights from outside with your curtains, invest in black out blinds or even a simple eye mask.

5) Turn off as many electrical appliances as possible, don't just leave them on standby. When some appliances are on standby they can use almost the same amount of electricity as they do when they are on and secondly the red light many of them have emits radiation which can interfere with your electromagnetic field. Everything connected to the Wifi and your mobile phones are all filling your room with frequencies while you sleep to, which aren't beneficial to your health.

If you use your phone to wake you up, invest in a battery-operated alarm clock to replace it or at the very least keep your devices far from your bed. You can also get a Himalayan crystal lamp in the room to absorb the frequencies while you sleep.

6) Switch to natural cotton bedding and naturally filled pillows (i.e. feather), which don't release low levels of toxins like synthetic materials do (i.e polyester).

7) Sleep without a pillow or only use one quite flat pillow to sleep with. Using a pile of pillows tilts our neck and takes our spine out of alignment which can cause neck and back problems.

Step 4 – Give a healthy makeover to at least 2 areas of your home this week

---

They can be areas of rooms instead of full rooms if time won't stretch to 2 full rooms.

So you can makeover your kitchen cupboards instead of your whole kitchen for example, which will probably inspire you to do the rest of your kitchen in the near future to match them.

To make this step a success, this week I am committed to:

_____

_____

_____

_____

_____

_____

_____

_____

_____

_____

_____

By the end of this week I hope to:

_____

_____

_____

_____

_____

Step 5 – **Affirmations**

I have used affirmations with clients and myself over the years to motivate, remind and inspire growth and change.

It can be challenging to make big changes in your life, especially if you are getting little support from those around you, this is where affirmations can be used very effectively. They can be the support you need to make it through.

One of the hardest changes I made in my life was to go raw vegan for a month, which doesn't seem that long now, but at the time it was a big deal.

I was about 3 months pregnant and concerned that it might not be the right time. I was worried that I couldn't handle such a change, I wondered if I should wait until the baby came and so on. But even with all these concerns, I really wanted to do it.

I decided to go for it, 100% raw and it felt great, I felt better than I did even before I got pregnant, all my so called pregnancy symptoms went.

But after about 10 days I was struggling to explain why I was doing it, to myself and others, so I wrote out the following affirmation:

Today I will be raw vegan because
It feels right
I don't want to be controlled by food anymore
I feel mentally stronger
I love all the energy I have
I am a good example to my family
I don't want to feel addicted
I don't want to make excuses for eating junk food
We were given every herb of the field as our meat
I can do it

I made several copies and stuck them up around my house and made sure that every time I saw it I'd read it to myself and I can't tell you how much it helped keep me on track.

It would always catch the eye of family, friends and even a salesmen that came to the house and they'd make some comment on it. I think it might have even inspired some of them to start looking at their own diet and lifestyle. I have used affirmations for my parenting, business and home schooling also.

Being at home with my children all day can be testing at the best of times, even though it's very rewarding.

There are times when I feel I'm not strong enough to continue with it all, I feel maybe the children would be better off in regular school, I feel that I am missing out on something by being at home all day and I get upset with myself for losing my temper sometimes with the children and myself. So to maintain some sanity and set me off on the right foot, I put this affirmation together some years ago

Today I will...
Be a loving mother to my children
Be a caring wife
Be patient
Work hard & stay focused
No shouting
No aggression
No quitting
Remember why you are doing this
To nurture, enrich & protect your family
Remember why you are here
To be the best you can be
Remember who you are
A mother, wife, Nuwaupian, teacher, protector

Here are some shorter affirmations that I use with my clients that you can add to your daily routine:

- I am nourished and fulfilled on every level
- I love being naturally me
- I have energy, happiness and abundant health
- Every cell in my body radiates bright beautiful health
- My sleep is relaxed and refreshing.
- I am healthy in body, mind and spirit
- I am strong, whole and healthy.
- I will stick to my eating plan and feel great for it
- I don't need alcohol / cigarettes / chocolate today because I already feel great
- I am glad to be working and will work with a smile today
- I will show kindness and caring to everyone I meet today
- I will accomplish my goals and fulfill my desires
- There is nothing I can not do
- Even though life is challenging, today will be a good day
- My journey is different from others but it's all mine
- Anything can be achieved when self doubt leaves

Step 5 – Use one of the above affirmations or make up your own that will help you achieve one of your health or life goals this week

Make sure you say it several times every day for a week.

See how close you are to achieving that goal or feeling better about life by the end of the week. Any progress will be an achievement.

To make this step a success, this week I am committed to:

_____

_____

_____

_____

_____

_____

_____

_____

_____

_____

By the end of this week I hope to:

_____

_____

_____

_____

Step 6 – Do What You Love

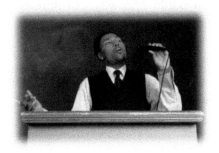

I once heard a song lyric that said *' If you find a job you love, you'll never work another day in your life'*

Hearing that put such a big smile on my face because after a few years of working in dead end jobs or pretty good jobs that I just didn't like, I have finally found the career that gives my life purpose and meaning, it actually nourishes me doing the work I do, I am so grateful for that.

Conversely, I know many people who are working jobs they hate and feel trapped because financially they currently believe they can't afford to quit.

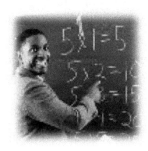

The reason we are addressing this here, is because you could be eating the best fresh organic foods that perfectly suits your body (more about this in Step 23), getting a good amount of exercise, avoiding cigarettes, alcohol and other drugs, making loads of money so you're able to afford the best of everything, but still feel terrible because your job is sucking the life out of you.

I've heard people describe their work as 'soul destroying', yet they stayed for the money. This is another way of subtly admitting that you have put a price on your soul and happiness, which are both priceless.

You could of course find work that is more fulfilling and rewarding to you. But in the meantime, you could find ways of making the best of a temporarily bad situation until you make the break. For example:

1. If you're a salesperson, don't just go to visit prospective clients at their office, invite them out to lunch, brunch or even drinks (to heck with the client services budget, it's there for a reason, use it)

2. If you don't wear a uniform to work, don't wear the same suit or clothes day in, day out. Wear your best clothes all the time, really make an effort with your clothes. It will make you feel special and you'll probably get treated differently by others too.

3. Let your voice be heard, if you don't like your work because of the way the company is being run, let your bosses know, they might even listen to you and make steps to improve the company which could make your work life easier to handle. If you feel you're voice won't be listened to, you won't know that until you try. If you fear speaking up will get you fired, you REALLY NEED TO MAKE PLANS TO LEAVE NOW.

4. Change things around. It's easy to fall into a routine at a job we've been at for a while, so change your routine as much as you can while still fulfilling your duties. Move your breaks around if you can, do your morning work in the afternoon, completely rearrange your desk, change the script you use, anything you can change, change.

5. If you're feeling bored in your work and you feel you could handle more work, ask for more responsibility, but be careful you don't get over burdened

Are you self- employed or a business owner?

Even when you take the great big juicy step of following your dreams and starting your own business, you can still end up not actually doing what you love and instead, becoming an employee in your own business. With so many facets of running a business, you can also find yourself fulfilling a role in your business that isn't suited to your passion and talents.

So you can be a great manager but a terrible marketer
You can be extremely creative but terrible at being organised
You can have a brilliant head for figures and creating profit but useless at creating the products

If you find yourself as an employee in your own business or carrying out a role in your business not suited to you, it can make the dream of being self employed or running a business turn into a nightmare.

Before this happens or if it's already happening, get your hands on the book "The E Myth" by Michael e Gerber and get reading.

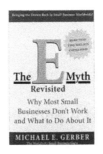

51

Becoming Naturally You

Have you found your path yet?

The idea of being at home all day with no great responsibilities or anywhere to rush off to on a cold winter morning can sound like bliss to some of us, but if this is your current situation because you haven't found your calling in life yet, then I'm guessing there's only so much of this life you'll be able to take before you want to find your path in life and begin to pursue it.

My brother, Julian Hall The Utlrapreneur has a simple tool he's devised to help you find a starting point or get an idea of the job, business or life that you can work towards that will make the best use of your skills and talents, that you are also driven to do.

The Success Equation

According to Julian:

"We've grown up being told that you've gotta be good at what you do or no one will employ you. Fair enough. We're also told that to be an entrepreneur you've gotta be passionate about what you do. Fair enough.

But no one ever told us that being good at what you do doesn't mean you're going to be passionate about it. Neither did they tell us that because you're passionate about something that you'll actually be any good at it.

So here goes:
The Ultrapreneurs Success Formula:

Passion + Excellence = Success

But how do you work out what you're passionate about and excellent at?

That's simple.

First grab a blank sheet of paper. On one side at the top write "Passion" and the other write "Excellence". Then make a list of what you're passionate about and a list of what you're excellent at.

Once the lists are complete, draw a line between key words that match, are similar or related in some way. Whatever that ends up being, and I mean whatever, that's what you should do with your life, in business or otherwise. "

When I did Julian's test, this is what showed up for me, which was great as it was all the things I currently do!!!

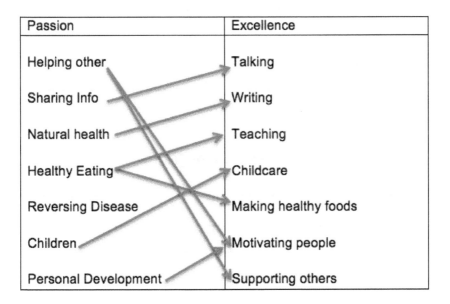

Passion	Excellence
Helping other	Talking
Sharing Info	Writing
Natural health	Teaching
Healthy Eating	Childcare
Reversing Disease	Making healthy foods
Children	Motivating people
Personal Development	Supporting others

Step 6 – Work out if you're doing what you love this week, if not, do something about it.

Really take some time this week to decide if what you spend your life doing, is what you love, if not make some real steps to find out what will bring you more joy and how best to attain it. Have a look at the action sheet at the end of this section related to this too.

To make this step a success, this week I am committed to:

_____

_____

_____

_____

_____

By the end of this week I hope to:

_____

_____

_____

_____

Step 7 – The Real Enemy

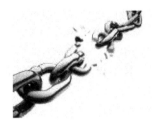

As much as we want to make an enemy out of the addictive foods we can't stop eating (or the companies that create them), the uncaring mean trainers at the gyms that train us unsympathetically, our job that doesn't pay us enough or the people around us who holds us back, there are 5 mindsets that many of us have that are the real enemies.

There are common thought patterns that have to be broken if you are going to achieve any goal you put your mind to.

Negative Associations

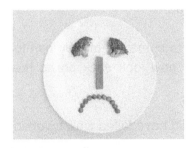

Experiences we go through, literally from birth, stay with us stored in our subconscious and can affect every decision we make. If you are struggling to achieve something, look at the dynamics of the situation, then look into your past to see if you've had negative experiences with the same thing in the past. This can take some time as the link may not be obvious.

For example, If you have personally failed on every diet you've ever tried, this can obviously make you less committed to any diet you take on in the future, but, less obviously, if your mother used to always be on a diet that was really restrictive and made her miserable, but still overweight and she often complained about it, this can also make YOU less likely to want to diet or expect it to be any different to your mother's experience.

Fear of Failure

This is the biggest and most common obstacle that stops someone achieving greatness. It's easier not to even bother trying than to try and fail right? Well if you train yourself to think like this, you might as well not get out of bed in the morning.

I heard a famous business success coach called Ali Brown say that she gets her clients to write down the five biggest achievements and greatest moments in their lives. Then she asks them if they had to sacrifice or do something they feared to achieve them and if they were easy to do.

Her clients realised that they did have to come out of their comfort zones to achieve the things that they now look back on as their greatest achievements.

There was a very real chance they could have failed whilst working to achieve them, but they didn't. Change the way you perceive a challenge, instead of worrying about whether you'll fail or not, look past that and focus on the benefits you can gain by deciding to go for it.

"Imagine what you'd be if you knew there was nothing you couldn't be"

Leah Salmon

Lack of Self Worth

The steps you take to improve yourself will normally involve an investment of your time, sometimes other people's time and your money. If you are discouraged to do something because it will take up people's time and it costs money, you are saying to yourself, those around you and the universe, that you're not worth a particular amount of money and time. This couldn't be further from the truth and you must never think like this.

There are practicalities that might mean you have to save up the money, organise your time and arrange child care for example, but if you decide you want something, whether it's a course, program, workshop, starting a business, pursuing a worthy and fulfilling new life path, or anything for that matter, make sure you get it because you are worth it and the people you feel you are "inconveniencing", could even be inspired by your drive to achieve your goal.

Laziness

"Tomorrow is the only day of the year that appeals to a lazy man" – Jimmy Lyons

57

Once you decide to do something, don't wait, act now. Be honest with yourself, if the only thing that is stopping you is sheer laziness, then you don't deserve the rewards available to you until you get out of your own way. If your laziness is induced by a poor diet or generally not taking care of your health, focus on Steps 12-29 to boost your health naturally, which will in turn help you regain your energy so you can start working on your goals.

Fear of Success
This concept can take some time to fully understand, but there are people out there who hit a ceiling in their growth and sometimes never even get off the ground because they are actually afraid of being successful. Everyone says they want money and success and power, but on a subconscious level we all realise that with great wealth comes great responsibility.

If you are used to relying on others to look after you (i.e. you live off state benefits, your partner makes all the money, your parents still look after you), once you have success financially, you'll possibly have to rely on yourself and lose the comfort of someone else being responsible for providing for you.

If you have always used your health condition as an excuse as to why you don't get out and socialise for example, once you change your diet and lifestyle and get well, you won't have that excuse to be antisocial anymore, so you'll be forced to admit the real reason you don't like going out and meeting new people.

If you used your weight as an excuse so you didn't have to go outside and play football with your children or do more with them, help more around the house etc, while you sit and watch the television, once you are shown a sure fire way to lose the weight, you lose your excuse and you'll have to admit the real reason you didn't want to be an active member of the family.

You get the sympathy vote when you have an illness or serious disease, people fall over themselves trying to help you, you can use it to get out of virtually anything you don't want to do. Once you consciously work towards improving your health, you'll lose your excuses.

Are you afraid you won't get the attention you did while you were ill? Or did you think that your illness made you interesting and special, so now you're well, you'll be ordinary and maybe even unremarkable? If you have always talked about all the people you are going to help and all the great things you are going to do when you make it big, when the opportunity comes along and you get that break, you are going to have to walk the walk that came with the big talk.

If any of the above fits you, then a good life coach or counsellor can help you get past the excuses that are hindering your growth so you can flourish and become Naturally You, sharing your skills and abilities with the whole world, which is what you are destined to do.

Step 7 – Identify if any of these blockages are present in you and work to remove them this week

---

Ask yourself "Are any of these mindsets blocking my success at attaining my health and life goals?" If so, find a way to start dealing with them this week. Seek help from a coach or mentor if needed.

To make this step a success, this week I am committed to:

_____

_____

_____

_____

_____

_____

_____

_____

_____

_____

By the end of this week I hope to:

_____

_____

_____

_____

_____

Step 8 – Social & Supported

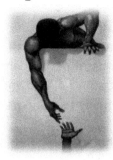

In the top 10 best selling book topics, diet and self improvement books and products are way up there with cookery books, autobiographies and books on Ancient Egipt. So if you want to change your life and your diet, you've got a lot of company.

Even so, it can still be a pretty lonely journey, especially when those you live and work with either don't understand what you're doing, think it's silly, strange or unnecessary.

But never fear, there's always someone out there going through the same challenges as you, you just need to find them and have a good old chin wag.

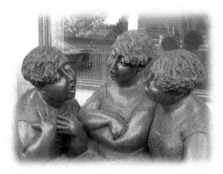

There are so many ways to socialise and network with other people who are into the same thing as you, who can provide an excellent support system during your journey of self and health discovery.

Here are a few suggestions of places to go to find fellow self developers:

The Internet & Social Networks: Without even leaving your armchair you can be connected with thousands of people who are doing the same thing as you. Even though I'd recommend physically going to networking events and actually meeting people,

I have connected with more people via the internet that have supported my growth, than I could have ever done networking one to one. Facebook, MeetUp, Twitter, Instagram and forums are great ways to meet big numbers of people and get lots of good information too.

Talks, Courses, Seminars and Workshops: Learning more about the new life you're pursuing can keep you focused and motivated. When I was starting my raw food journey early in one of my pregnancies, I decided to finally go on a one day 'Raw Food For Beginners' class I'd been looking at for some time.

I was excited to go because of what I'd learn, but when I got there I found that for the first time ever, I was actually in a room with 20 other people who enjoyed raw food as much as I did.   They'd either experienced eating a raw diet or were very keen on trying it, so I could share my experiences with them and they could relate.

I left that course with a stack of information and practical tips and a renewed energy that kept me going for months.

Big Events and Exhibitions: These events normally attract the big names in their field, so you'll get the social interaction of the visitors, exhibitors, stall holders and staff, but also talks from accomplished professionals in your field of interest. Exhibitors trying to get their products out there are also likely to give out free samples, tasters and discounts on their products and services too, especially in the health field. I come home with a whole bag of freebies and vouchers when I go to them!!!!

Coaching Programs: Individual or small group coaching is a more intimate and focused way to succeed in your chosen journey. A good coach can help you identify potential problems before they arise so you are equipped to deal with them before they interfere with your progress.

Gyms, Studios, Health Stores - Your local gym, health studio or health store should have information on local events and specialists you can go and see. The staff themselves can be a good source of information and inspirational too.

Step 8 – Commit to going to one new place to get social support this week, go there this week if possible too

Find places you can go to meet like-minded people whilst gaining more knowledge about the new lifestyle you've chosen to follow.

If it's a physical event, send out a message to your friends with the event details to find out if anyone wants to come with you, you may find you already have a group of fellow self-developers without even leaving your circle of friends.

To make this step a success, this week I am committed to:

_____

_____

_____

_____

_____

_____

_____

_____

_____

_____

_____

By the end of this week I hope to:

_____

_____

_____

_____

_____

Step 9 – Colour Therapy

Different colours have different energies and the ability to affect our health, moods and environment. You can use coloured clothes and objects to help you achieve your health goals while enriching your environment.

Take a look around your home and wardrobe for a moment, how do the colours of things (or lack of them) make you feel? Have you noticed that nothing around you is in your favourite colour? Do the colours of your walls, bedding, clothes, shoes, table mats, underwear, rugs and cushions bringing a smile to your face and nourish your being or are they just whatever colour you could find at the time?

There are many schools of thought on what different colours represent and you can even find out which colours work of you personally, but here are some interpretations of colours you can use when deciding what colours to add to your life:

Red excites, warms, stimulates and encourages movement

Orange is energising and can help reduce fatigue and tiredness, If you get bored with your work, put a bright orange object on your desk or work space.

Yellow is an energising colour like the rays of the sun. If you want to remember something, jot it down on yellow paper (remember the original Post it Notes were all pale yellow). It can also help relieve depression.

Green is closely associated with nature, it promotes healing on many levels and encourages emotional and psychological balance

Blue is calming, relaxing and can help cool you down. Big pictures of the beach with the blue water and sky can help bring calmness to a room.

Pink can help tranquilise aggression, which is why it's used in prisons, hospitals and juvenile centres. It's also a good colour for the bedroom as it promotes love and affection.

Black represents supreme balance, beauty, control and power. Wear black if you want to feel strength and self confidence.

Different shades and brightness of colour can also effect their properties, but as all colours can have a positive effect somehow, finding a colour that truly resonates with you is a great way to choose.

Step 9 – Introduce 3 new colours to your life this week

This can be in your clothes, shoes, coats, jewellery (which is where I normally include it), bedding, sofa cushions, curtains, hand bag, plates, cups, table clothes, towels and more, anywhere you can.

To make this step a success, this week I am committed to:

_____

_____

_____

_____

_____

_____

_____

_____

_____

_____

_____

By the end of this week I hope to:

_____

_____

_____

_____

_____

Step 10 – Vision Board Your Goals

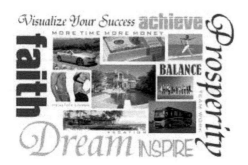

Vision boards are a fun way of keeping focused on your goals and making your goals a visual part of your environment.

When you look at it, it has to be able to almost instantly remind you of the things you want to have and achieve. So when creating it, put a lot of thought into it and find pictures that fit your aspirations as closely as possible. So don't just find a picture of any sports car, find a picture of the exact make and model you dream about.

Don't just get a picture of a big house, find a picture of a house you can see yourself living in once you're making the big bucks! If you want to exercise more, add a picture of something that will remind you of fitness (hands weights, a gym, skipping rope, someone stretching, trainers etc). If you want to eat more salads, find a picture of a big juicy appetising salad. If you want to spend more time with your partner, add a picture of where you'd like to spend time with them. You can cut out words that go with your dream too.

Flick through some newspapers and magazines and cut out the images you need. You might need to draw on it, stick other things on it and rearrange the pictures and words a few times until it's perfect.

You can create your whole vision board digitally if you want, search Google images for pictures, use pictures you've taken and uploaded to your computer or tablet, then create it all in a Microsoft Word document and print it out.

When it's ready, hang it up somewhere you can see it daily. Just like with the affirmations, the more you see if, the closer you get to attaining those goals.

My brother Julian Hall The Ultrapreneur also has a saying in his book "Entrepreneur to Ultrapreneur – 100 Ways To Up Your Game" that says, "Vision boards mean nothing if your vision doesn't make sense", so following the advice above will make sure you're more likely to create a vision board that's aligned to you and therefore easier for you to achieve.

Step 10 – Make a vision board this week

You can get started by looking for the best images in magazines, online or old photos you have, then find the words you want to add if any and get to work.

If you're making a physical one, grab a large piece of paper, card or a corkboard, some scissors, pins, sticky tape or glue and your pictures and words. If you're making it digitally, get your device in hand. Either way, find a time you can work undisturbed for about and hour, get some snacks and a drink, put some music on and go for it.

Remember, it can be full to the brim with gorgeous words and images or sparse with just a few pictures and words, it's entirely up to you.

To make this step a success, this week I am committed to:

_____

_____

_____

_____

_____

_____

_____

_____

_____

_____

_____

By the end of this week I hope to:

_____

_____

_____

_____

_____

Step 11 – Bribery & Corruption

Many practitioners and health coaches won't agree with this approach, but in certain circumstances, when willpower alone isn't getting the results, you need to resort to a few under hand tactics.

There are times we literally need to be saved from ourselves, we know we want to make changes, but we also realise that temptation can be our downfall. So offering ourselves rewards for good behaviour and making sure there's no way we can cheat, can get the results we desire. Some examples of this are:

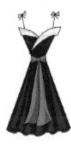 **The Perfect Dress** - I got one of my clients to buy the dress she'd been talking about for weeks, but in a dress size below the one she was at the time. We set up a goal that she would get down to that dress size by a certain date, and if she did, she could wear that dress out on the town.

She kept the dress (which cost a pretty penny) hung outside her wardrobe as a constant reminder of her goal. You could do the same with a suit to wear to a big event.

Find Someone To Nag You - Tell everyone around you what you're doing and give them all explicit permission to have a go at you if they catch you back sliding. The best people to tell are people you're likely to see daily who love to tell you what to do anyway.

If you're the type of person that doesn't like being told what to do, this may not be the best tactic for you (your poor friend who follows your instruction might get their head bitten off), but if you can handle advice, this can turn your quest for health and happiness into a family affair.

Leave Yourself No Choice - I found that every time I went out, whether I was actually hungry or not, if I had money I'd buy junk, especially sweet things and chocolates. So when I switched to a sugar free diet, I found the best strategy was to leave all my money at home so I had nothing to spend.

I was working in a hospital at the time, so I bought a weekly travel card to get on public transport and a packed lunch of foods I could eat and my mobile phone in case of an emergency and that was it.

Make A Financial Commitment - If you're the type of person who doesn't like to waste money, pay for several months of gym membership or the services of a personal trainer up front so that you are more inclined to use it.

For some, this won't work, once they've spent the money they simply forget about it. For others, the more they invest, the more likely they are to show up, on time, do what's asked of them and get the results.

Get Some Help - I was finding it so hard to control my love of chocolate (I was eating it more than once a day sometimes) I had to enlist the help of my husband. I gave him 5 bars of chocolate, asked him to hide them so I couldn't find them, then he could give me small amounts when I asked for some, but no more than once a day or every other day. I asked him to check that when I went out I didn't take any money with me and it worked great, within 2 weeks the daily cravings had gone and I felt so much better.

Step 11 – If you really need to, use one of the above or another incentive that will help you stick to your goals.

To make sure it's going to work for the whole length of the program, it's fine to change the incentive along the way if the current one becomes less desirable or effective. Once you achieve a goal and get your reward, set another one with another reward to keep you on your toes, always striving to create a better you.

To make this step a success, this week I am committed to:

_____

_____

_____

_____

_____

_____

By the end of this week I hope to:

_____

_____

_____

Your Becoming Naturally You Mind & Environment Action Sheets

Are You Doing What You Love?

In Step 6 we spoke about finding a job or life path you love or finding ways of making your current work more enjoyable. There are so many ways to make a clean break from a job you hate if you really wanted to. It would take courage, focus and determination, but it is possible. This exercise is to compare your current and desired life. It could be the motivation you need to make the break and it can show you the life you want so you can start living it now.

Give yourself a whole hour for this exercise. In the table below (use more paper if you run out of space), write down all the things you love and dislike about your job or current life. If you are unemployed, write about you current income wherever it comes from (benefit, support from a partner etc) and current lifestyle.

Before you start writing, give yourself a few minutes to think about a few typical days, good and bad. Read over everything you've written a few times.

On the next page, you are going to describe your dream job or life, don't hold anything back here, let it all out, be as creative, adventurous and ambitious as you can.

Compare the 2 sheets and decide whether you're living the dream already, or still dreaming about living. It's time to start living.

Your Current Job / Life Path

My name is _____

And I work / spend my time

_____

Things I love about my current job / life	Things I dislike about my current job / life

My Wage / Salary / Income is _____ a year / month

I work _____ hours a day, _____ days a

week , _____ weeks a year.

I have been working in this job / following this life path for:
_____ weeks / months / years

In that time, the progress I've made in my life and career is:

This Is My Dream Job / life

My name is _____

And I work / spend my days

_____

I work _____ days a week, _____ hours a day

My (work) day normally starts at _____ and finishes at

_____

I earn _____ a month after tax

I take _____ weeks holiday a year

(*If you're not self employed or a business owner*) My bonuses include (*i.e.* company car):

_____

_____

_____

I work/live in (*state town and country*)
_____ which I love

I get to spend _____ hours / days with my
loved ones every _____

I have _____ hours / days to spend personally,
professional, emotionally, mentally developing myself every

_____

The best things about this job/life are

1.

2.

3.

Take a **GOOD** look around you?

It's time to stop and smell the roses. This task is about identifying the positive things in your environment and spending some time appreciating them.

In the box below, write all the things you can think of, under the titles given, that make you feel good, motivate your growth, keep you on track, show you love and understanding and generally are good to be around.

Once you have finished, read over them and in whatever way feels right to you, thank, bless or acknowledge them for being there. We are given many gifts and blessings in life and the best thing we can do to show appreciation for them, is to first recognise they are there.

I am grateful for and love...	
Family Members	
Friends	

Foods/Drinks Natural Remedies	
Places	
Books, Information Products, websites	
Clothes/ Shoes/ Jewellery	
Physical Activities	
Other Things	

Your Becoming Naturally You Food Steps

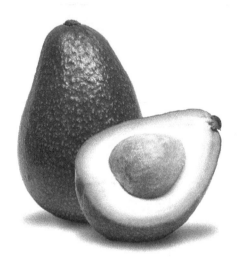

"A generation on whole foods will turn hospitals into museums"

Leah Salmon

Among other things, it was the quote from Hippocrates that said "If doctors of today don't become nutritionists, the doctors of tomorrow will be nutritionist" that made me decide to dedicate my life to learning, studying and trying to help others with their food and diet when I first started.

It gave me visions of patients in the future leaving the doctor's surgery with a genuine smile on their faces, not because the doctor's just cracked a cheesy joke while he handed them a prescription for one of their favourites (Paracetamol, antibiotics or steroids), but because they had finally found a real answer to their problems.

All too often my clients tell me how their doctors gave them a clean bill of health yet they still felt terrible. Then, with sometimes very few dietary amendments, together we manage to get rid of their symptoms. This phenomenon is becoming more commonplace and the concept of using your food as your medicine is not as wild as it sounds.

Sometimes a suggestion sounds too simple to be effective, until you try it and find it works.

We eat everyday and some of us eat an awful lot every day, so it stands to reason that looking at what you eat is a good place to start if you want to improve your health is some way. Along side their area of expertise, many other complementary therapists are now giving some type of dietary advice to their clients as it's benefits can't be ignored.

They know that if the herbs, aromatherapy, exercises or practices they prescribe them are being given to a junk food eating, alcohol drinking, 20–a-day smoking body, they're far less likely to get the results they should do.

Your food can do so much more for you than just taste nice. It can give you energy, improve your moods, get rid of common complaints like headaches, colds, aches and pains, help you lose, gain or maintain weight and muscle mass and even improve your love life and most importantly your love *of* life.

So now that we got your mind and environment to a nourished and supportive place, lets look at 18 weekly steps you can take with your food that will get you to love your life.

Step 12 – The Three Nasties

There are 3 phrases that will send shivers up any nutritionist's spine and they are:

Monosodium Glutamate
Aspartame
Trans Fatty Acids

These are possibly the biggest failures of science and man in the last millennia. To fully explain the extent to which these three contribute to bad health would take three whole books, but in short here's a bit about them.

Monosodium Glutamate

- **What is it?** MSG is short for MonoSodium Glutamate, which is also known as a flavour enhancer and a meat tenderiser.
- **Where is it?** This chemical comes in a white powder form and is found in savoury foods like crisps, burgers, soup mixes, frozen foods, processed food and is very popular in Chinese take away and junk food.
- **What does it do?** MSG consumption can lead to stomach cramps, nausea, depression, mood swings, insomnia, runny nose, blurred vision, joint pains, headaches, inflamed tongue and more. This dangerous compound actually makes you crave more of it once you've eaten it, which is why the slogan 'once you pop you can't stop' is so fitting.

Aspartame

- **What is it?** It's reported to be 200 times sweeter than sugar so manufacturers can sweeten their products for much less than the cost of sugar, but at the expense of our health. It's made of 3 poisons – Phenylalanine, Aspartic acid and Methanol/wood alcohol, which on their own cause enough damage.
- **Where is it?** This drug cocktail is found in about 5000 products. It is a common replacement for sugar in diet and sugar free slimming and diabetic products, but it's also found in sweets, cakes, chewing gum, fizzy drinks, jams, sauces, jellies and a whole host of fast foods.
- **What does it do?** There are reportedly 92 adverse conditions that are associated with the consumption of aspartame including muscle spasms, weight gain, rashes, depression, fatigue, irritability, memory loss and joint pain.

Trans Fatty Acids /Hydrogenated Oils

- **What is it?** This substance is produced when liquid vegetable oils are hardened at room temperature to create products like margarine, through a process called hydrogenation. It basically extends the shelf life of oils and gives the manufacturer more ways to add them to your food.
- **Where is it?** Trans fats are found in processed junk foods, crisps, cakes, biscuits, sauces, soups, breads, crackers, sweets, ready meals, margarine, shortening etc.
- **What does it do?** It can prevent the uptake of essential fatty acids, increase weight, dry your skin, increase cholesterol levels, affect a diabetics response to insulin, promote heart disease, cancer, obesity and reproductive problems.

84

Step 12 - Don't eat or drink anything with MSG, Aspartame & Trans Fats for 7 days

The best way to do this is to make a list of everything in your cupboards, fridge, freezer and pantry that has any of these on the label, then next to each item write down an alternative you can use or buy to replace that item and then throw that item away, it's such a liberating feeling to be so bold with this.

So for example, if you have margarine in the fridge, put it on your list, write something like "real butter" or "trans fat free spread" next to it and then bin the margarine.

If you have soya sauce with MSG you could write Tamari or miso next to it and then bin the soya sauce.

And if you have bottles of drinks with aspartame in them, you could write fresh homemade juice or water next to it then bin the bottle.

If you need to take things more slowly because too much of your food has these ingredients, remove one at a time, so first remove and replace all the foods with MSG, then trans or hydrogenated fats, then aspartame.

Unopened food can be donated to a local food bank if you prefer not to waste them by throwing them out.

To make this step a success, this week I am committed to:

_____

_____

_____

_____

_____

_____

_____

_____

_____

_____

_____

_____

By the end of this week I hope to:

_____

_____

_____

_____

_____

Step 13 – Wonderful Water

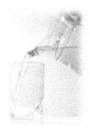

Why drinking enough water is so important

Depending on your size and height, your body can use up to 2 ½ litres every day, just to carry out simple functions like digestion and cleansing.

If you don't supply your body with fresh clean water on a daily basis, guess what? Your body will draw water out of your bones, eyes, skin and other organs to carry out its functions. Dehydration signs could be anything from headaches and bad skin to dark yellow urine and constipation.

Drink first when you get hungry

According to Dr F Batmanghelidj on page 93 of his award winning best seller 'Your Body's Many Cries For Water' it states,

'The front of the brain either gets energy from 'hydroelectricity' (a water pump system) or from sugar in the blood circulation'

'…sensations of thirst and hunger are generated simultaneously to indicate the brain's needs. We do not recognise the sensations of thirst and assume both to be indicators of the urge to eat. (So) we eat food even when our body should receive water.'

Therefore, my advice would be to always drink a glass of water when you get a hunger pang. If the hunger pain is still there 10 minutes later then go for a healthy snack or a meal if it's near a meal time. If the hunger pang is gone after 10 minutes, drink some more water to be sure you've fulfilled your body's current need.

Don't drink with meals

If you drink with or just after your meals, it's probably because your meals don't naturally have a high enough water content or you are dehydrated through the day.

When you eat, your body needs water to digest food, so if you haven't had enough water in the day, your body will call for it just to help digest your food.

When your body senses foods, it releases acidic digestive juices to fully breakdown the food, so once it's been chewed properly, then the juices get to work before sending it to your bowels.

When you drink with your meals in large amounts, you dilute or wash out these juices so your food doesn't get broken down properly and is sent to your bowels in clumps. In this state, the nutrients in the food are inaccessible and can't be absorbed by the body.

This whole process leads to gas, bloating, food sensitivities and worst of all, you not getting all the nutrients you could from the foods you spend your hard earned money on.

By drinking regularly throughout the day, 20 minutes before or 1 hour after you eat, you avoid this whole palaver. Including a big green or fresh vegetable salad with your meals will also make you less likely to want to drink, while providing a natural lubricating refreshing element to your meals.

Jazz Up Your Cup

If you don't like the taste of water, here are 3 things you can try to make it more palatable

1. Add a pinch of salt – This can make it taste more mouth like so it's easier to drink. It also helps your body to absorb the water so you're not going to the toilet too frequently. Use a pinch of salt to a 2 litre bottle of water and give it a good shake. Don't worry, you won't even taste it.

2. Add a squeeze of lemon – This can give the water a little flavour without adding too much sugar and it's a cleansing and alkalising drink too.

3. Drink it at room temperature – When you drink cold water, it can put a shock on your internal organs. Your body needs to burn calories to increase the temperature of the water to body temperature before it can absorb it. But drinking water at room temperature makes it easier on your body and for some, it tastes better too.

Glass over Plastic

When it comes to storing your water, aim to store it in glass bottles. Most plastic bottles will leach their chemicals into the water in tiny amounts over time. These chemicals are harmful to our endocrine and nervous system, even if we are only taking in tiny amounts at a time. You can get bottles made of a plastic that's safer to drink from, described as **2HDPE** or BPA free, so get these if you don't want to use glass.

I found that washing out and reusing big molasses, olive and honey jars was a great way to create lots of glasses and glass water storage bottle instead of buying them.

Step 13 - Follow the 4 water rules above for 7 days

Institute this simple daily water routine, which is easy to remember:

Make sure you have
2 glasses of water when you wake up
2 more before lunch,
2 more before dinner
& 2 more 1 hour before bed

If you currently drink less than 4 glasses a day you can start by having just one glass at these times, then increase it to 1 ½ then 2. Spreading them out even more is optimal but this is a good start

Drinking more water will become a habit that your body will start to remind you to do once you become well hydrated again, It does get easier, trust me.

To make this step a success, this week I am committed to:

_____

_____

_____

_____

_____

_____

_____

_____

_____

_____

By the end of this week I hope to:

_____

_____

_____

_____

_____

Step 14 – Get Those Juices Flowing

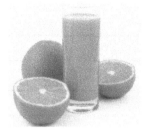

I was shocked to learn while writing this book, that as well as all the sugar, preservatives and other unnatural additives they put into cartons of commercially produced fruit and vegetable juices, most of them are also pasteurised, which means they are boiled to increase their shelf life and remove impurities.

So the live enzymes that you would get from freshly made juices would all be destroyed once boiled, In saying that, it's also true that if you leave a freshly made juice to stand for more than 20 minutes a certain amount of the nutrients in it will have died off anyway. So the benefits of freshly made juices are highest when they are drunk shortly after juicing.

The difference between and juice and a smoothie, is that a juice is made by taking fruit and veg and either blending them and straining them or putting them through a juicer, which separates the juice from the fibres which is called pulp. A smoothie is made by simply liquefying fruit and veg in a blender then drinking the whole lot.

Michael Van Straten, whose book "Super Juice" helped me to successfully finish my very first 5 day juice feast with incredible results, says

'Juicing is the fool-proof way of adding wonderful life-giving, life-enhancing and life-protecting vitamins, minerals and natural food chemicals to your diet. Sure, you could take pills, but they contain only the nutrients we know about in artificial form. On the other hand, the nutrients in fresh juice are more easily absorbed by the body. What's more it contains trace elements, vitamins and minerals that scientists are only just beginning to discover'.

That sounds like a good enough reason to get juicing to me. Before you start juicing, here are some suggestions to make them even better for you

1. Always dilute juices with water, especially fruit juices which can be very sweet
2. Vegetables like broccoli, spinach, kale and fresh herbs add a lot of nutrition but very little actually juice comes from these particular veggies.
3. Juicy fruits and vegetables like cucumbers, celery, oranges, apples and even carrots, give you a lot more juice, if you want a larger drink.
4. Berries don't make a lot of juice at all, but taste great blended into a freshly made juice.
5. Bananas and avocados are examples of fruits that can't be juiced as they have no water. Again, these can be blended into a fresh juice.
6. Even though its best to drink a juice straight away, to save time, you can store it in the fridge for about a day without it going off or losing excessive amounts of nutrients. Adding lemon to your juices can help preserve it also.

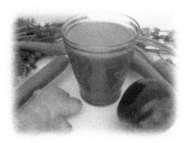

93

There are tons of juice recipes out there, but here are a few to get you started:

- Apple and carrot
- Cucumber, celery, apple
- Orange, beetroot and carrot
- Spinach, cucumber, apple and coriander
- Raspberry, apple and orange
- Celery, spinach, lemon, apple
- Pineapple, orange and apple
- Redcurrant, apple, lemon & ginger
- Pear, apple and ginger
- Beetroot, celery, cucumber and carrot
- Lettuce, apple, celery and lemon
- Spinach, celery and apple

Step 14 - Treat yourself to a different juice for a week

Use the tips given in this step and start off with simple recipes like those given above or combinations of your favourite fruits and vegetables.

You can find out what fruits and vegetables are in season, using the chart in Step 18 of this book.

If you haven't already done the Healthy Home Makeover of your kitchen as mentioned in Step 4, you may want to at least look over that step to get your kitchen ready to start juicing daily.

To make this step a success, this week I am committed to:

_____

_____

_____

_____

_____

_____

_____

_____

_____

_____

_____

By the end of this week I hope to:

_____

_____

_____

_____

_____

Step 15 – There Are No Teeth In Your Tummy

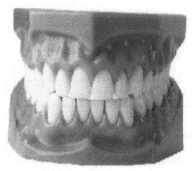

In Chinese medicine and with some of my own clients, looking at the tongue can be a great tool in finding out the general health of their body.

A very famous nutritionist once did a talk in which a man stood up and asked her to look at his tongue. She was fascinated because it was the clearest tongue she'd ever seen, almost like a baby's. A tongue that is clear, with no patches in the coating, spots or red, black or yellow markings is a sign of a pretty healthy body.

She asked him what diet he was on and how old he was. The whole room was shocked that he was 70 years old as he only looked about 50. Even more surprising was that he had never been on any diet. He ate what he wanted whenever he wanted, but for his whole life he had always chewed his food until it was a liquid consistency, which he had learned from his grandmother. He claimed he had only had a few short lived colds in his life and no major illnesses.

Fully chewing your food breaks it down so that your body can actually get all the nutrients from it. When we swallow half chewed food, as there are no teeth in our tummies, (believe it or not) the nutrients can't be absorbed and so will pass out of us having done nothing but aggravate our system. There are African cultures who are reputed to chew each mouthful of food no less than 72 times!!!

Now, as you can imagine, or as you'll find out if you try it, this can be a long process, but life is geared to doing everything on the run, so junk food that requires 2 chews before swallowing fits right in with that.

Raw foods and whole foods require a certain amount of mastication. But the longer you chew, the more digestive juices that are produced in the mouth and the stomach to fully break your food down so you get the most from it.

An old saying I taught my children recently is "Drink your foods and chew your drinks", which emphasises the importance of chewing everything to get the nutrients from it, and at times you will literally see us chewing mouthfuls of green smoothie or chocolate milk a few times before swallowing!!!!

Step 15 - Chew one meal a day perfectly this week

Make a slightly smaller portion of one meal a day and chew each mouthful at least 30 times.   Try this for a week and see if you still feel as full and satisfied as you normally do with a regular sized portion.

Also notice how different food tastes when you chew it completely and see if there's any improvement to any digestive complaints you currently have.

To make this step a success, this week I am committed to:

_____

_____

_____

_____

_____

_____

_____

_____

_____

_____

_____

By the end of this week I hope to:

_____

_____

_____

_____

_____

_____

Step 16 – A Whole Lot Better

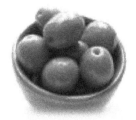

When foods grow in nature, they are in their complete whole form and with very little preparation, humans can eat them: most nuts just need to be taken out of their shells and herbs, fruits and vegetables just need to be washed and sometimes peeled.

Even simply steaming or cooking foods in water or by fire is as much as some foods need. Other foods can be fermented, dried out or soaked and sprouted to make them edible or more flavoursome.

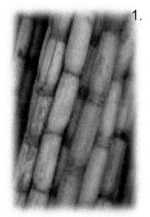

1. Foods in their whole state have the most nutrients in the forms of essential fatty acids, oils, fibre, vitamins, minerals, trace elements and if kept raw, live enzymes and phytonutrients too. When you pick sweetcorn from the field, remove the leaves, pick the kernels off, dry and mill them into maize or corn starch, then process them into corn syrup and add enzymes that turn it into High Fructose Corn Syrup, you've taken a whole natural quite health giving food into a dangerously sweet unnatural cheap additive, which some scientists claim is as addictive as cocaine.

The early 1900's saw the dawn of the industrial revolution; things could be done with foods that weren't previously dreamed of. Food processing methods were being developed that increased the shelf life of foods, supposedly made them taste better and most importantly enabled manufacturers to produce them for pennies instead of pounds. This has resulted in the highly refined and processed foods we have today.

Things like white sugar were at one time something only the very rich could afford, now you can buy 1kg of white sugar for 20p in some supermarkets. White flour can be bought for 11p and you can get 1 litre of vegetable oil for 80p.

Let's take a look at 3 of the white poisons plaguing our food chain today:

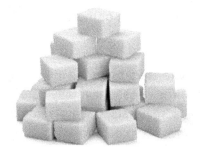

White sugar
White sugar is the most refined version of sugar, so all the nutrients are taken from it. It's highly addictive and it leaches nutrients from your body when you ingest it, which will make you vitamin and mineral deficient.

It can lead to type II diabetes, it feeds bacteria in your body allowing them to overgrow and cause horrible symptoms (e.g. candida, athlete's foot, etc.) and it can suppress the immune system making it easier for you to get sick, become infected and delay recovery from illnesses too. This is definitely not an exhaustive list of its dangers, but a start.

It can be found in a vast number of products including sweets, cakes, cereals, fast foods, pizza, herb seasonings, soups, ketchup, ready meals, yoghurts and chewing gums.

It can be replaced with:
Coconut sugar
Maple syrup (good quality and not mixed with sugar syrup)
Honey
Stevia
Molasses
Xylitol
Date sugar or paste
Very ripe bananas (to sweeten a cake or smoothies)

White Oils
White oils are mainly vegetable oils that are sold in clear plastic bottles with a pale yellow colour, which have been heated, deodorised, de gummed and combined with harmful chemicals like hexane, all of which remove the nutrients from the oils, making them rancid. These can be found in sweets, crisps, crackers, ready made meals, soups, sauces, junk food, pizza, chips and most food sold in fast food restaurants.

They can be replaced with:
Extra virgin olive oil
Virgin coconut oil
Unrefined palm oil
Ghee
Butter

There are other healthier oils, but don't just use them for cooking, for example flaxseed oil isn't meant to be heated but you can drizzle it over foods once they've been cooked to enhance their flavour, texture and nutritional content. We'll go into a lot more detail on oils and how best to use them in Step 26.

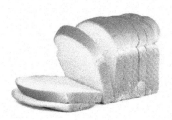

White Wheat flour
The refining process that wheat goes through removes virtually all the nutrients leaving you with a nutrient-dead, fibreless powder. It is so void of nutrition that the authorities in the USA & UK felt the need to add synthetic minerals and vitamins to it once processed to justify putting it on shelves for human consumption. Wholemeal flour has slightly more nutrients than white flour but not a great deal.

All wheat flours contain a protein called gluten, which in recent years has been found to cause a whole host of digestive and even psychological issues from weight gain, gut inflammation, constipation, IBS, fatigue and more. Gluten & wheat free diets have been found to help sufferers of everything from acne, and depression to PMS and infertility.

Whilst there is gluten found in other grains like barley, rice and spelt, the type of gluten found in wheat, coupled with the other properties of the much tampered with wheat plant of today, make wheat gluten more problematic than others. I've found that my children and other people I've worked with can tolerate the grains spelt, rye and rice to a degree, which all contain gluten, but they have an almost immediate reaction to wheat. You can find many other white flours today made from different grains or foods other than wheat, not all of them contain gluten and some haven't even been highly processed to become white, that's their natural colour, like potato and tapioca flour.

White wheat flour can be found in bread, cakes, biscuits, sauces, pasta, noodles, pizza bases, pies and pastries.

It can be replaced with:
Spelt flour
Coconut flour
Rye flour
Buckwheat flour
Brown rice flour

Wheat and gluten have particular properties that create soft spongy breads, cakes, pastries and pastas that hold together very easily (think of the word glue in gluten), which other flours don't all have. So it's best to find recipes that use these flours so you can use them to make alternatives that turn out properly, as sometimes you need to do more than just swap ingredients to get a good result. I've had some disastrous attempts at using other flours to make pancakes, breads and cakes in the past.

Step 16 - Replace all white wheat flour, sugar and oil products with their wholesome alternative for a week

---

If you need to stretch this step out over 3 weeks so that you replace one at a time, do that, if you use a lot of each, changing all of them at once might be quite a big overhaul, however if you're up for it, go for it!

To make this step a success, this week I am committed to:

_____

_____

_____

_____

_____

_____

_____

_____

_____

_____

By the end of this week I hope to:

_____

_____

_____

_____

_____

Step 17 – Get It Fresh & Local

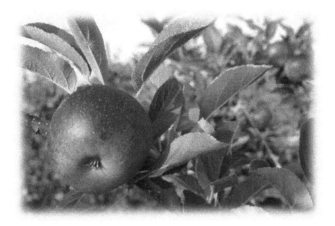

Why eat fresh foods

What's the biggest difference between a cooked meal made from fresh vegetables and one made from processed ones? It's true that a meal made from fresh produce often tastes better, but the amount of nutrition they give us is the biggest difference, but not something we can easily differentiate, which is another reason to cook most of our meals from scratch ourselves, to be more sure the ingredients are fresh and more nutrient rich.

From the moment a fruit or vegetable is picked it starts to lose nutrients. Nuts and seeds can become rancid over long periods of time and even water gets stagnant if left on the shelf for too long.

Processed foods are designed to have long shelf lives by manufacturers adding artificial substances that can prolong their appearance, smell, taste and texture, sometimes for years.

When a carrot is going off, you can see, taste, smell and feel the natural change it goes through. Processing foods halts that natural process and gives you the illusion of eating something that has all the benefits of its natural state.

Some forms of processing, like dehydrating, pickling, fermenting, and in some instances freezing, can preserve the nutrients (fermenting can even add more nutrients to the food), but there's nothing like getting food the way nature made it, without the processing to artificially maintain the appearance of freshness.

What's the point of eating locally produced foods?
The 2 biggest benefits of eating local produce, especially if you get it from a farmers' market, are the seasonality and the nutrient density of the food.

Farmers' markets (in the UK at least) are only allowed to sell produce that was grown within 100 miles of the market's location, This ensures to some degree that the produce you are getting is relatively fresh, not having been shipped or flown in from a country 1000's of miles away. So it's likely to be fresher and more nutrient dense

Farmers markets typically only sell seasonal produce, which means that, again, it's highly likely that it was grown naturally without the need for heat lamps or chemicals to encourage it to grow out of season.

As well as these benefits you may even get to speak to the farmers or producer of the food to find out what fertiliser they use, how their animals are kept and what they are fed. In general, food stores are beginning to realise just how important these kinds of things are to consumers and seem to actually make an effort to show you what they do with your food before you get it.

At farmers markets and farm shops, by speaking to the staff you can get a great deal of information about your food, from what's in season to the best recipe for homemade chicken burgers according to one of my sisters!!!

Step 17 - Have a "Fresh & Local Food" week.

Aim to eat all your fruit, vegetables, nuts, seeds and grains in their whole state, instead of the ready made, pre cooked, canned frozen or packaged varieties and aim to buy as much of it as you can from local sources like farmers markets, organic box schemes, farm shops, food co ops or local producers.

"Fertility clinics replaced orphanages when fast food replaced fresh food"

Leah Salmon

To make this step a success, this week I am committed to:

_____

_____

_____

_____

_____

_____

_____

_____

_____

_____

By the end of this week I hope to:

_____

_____

_____

_____

_____

Step 18 – Know Your Seasons

Produce	JAN	FEB	MAR	APR	MAY	JUN	JUL	AUG	SEP	OCT	NOV	DEC
APPLES, BRAMLEY							JUL	AUG	SEP			
APPLES, COX										OCT		
ASPARAGUS					MAY	JUN						
BEANS, BROAD						JUN	JUL	AUG				
BEANS, RUNNER							JUL	AUG	SEP	OCT		
BLACKBERRIES									SEP	OCT		
BLUEBERRIES							JUL	AUG	SEP			
BRUSSELS SPROUTS	JAN	FEB							SEP	OCT	NOV	DEC
CABBAGE, SPRING GREEN	JAN	FEB	MAR	APR				AUG	SEP	OCT	NOV	DEC
CABBAGE, WHITE									SEP	OCT	NOV	DEC
CABBAGE, SAVOY	JAN	FEB	MAR				JUL	AUG	SEP	OCT	NOV	DEC
CABBAGE, RED								AUG	SEP	OCT	NOV	
CARROTS	JAN	FEB				JUN	JUL	AUG	SEP	OCT	NOV	DEC
CAULIFLOWER	JAN	FEB	MAR	APR	MAY		JUL	AUG	SEP	OCT	NOV	DEC
CELERY							JUL	AUG	SEP	OCT		
CHERRIES							JUL	AUG				
COURGETTE						JUN	JUL	AUG	SEP			
CUCUMBER				APR	MAY	JUN	JUL	AUG	SEP			
KALE	JAN	FEB	MAR	APR					SEP	OCT	NOV	DEC
LEEKS	JAN	FEB	MAR						SEP	OCT	NOV	DEC
LETTUCE, COS							JUL	AUG	SEP			
LETTUCE, CURLY					MAY	JUN	JUL	AUG				
LETTUCE, ICEBERG							JUL	AUG	SEP			
MARROW								AUG	SEP	OCT		
PEAS						JUN	JUL	AUG	SEP			
PLUMS								AUG	SEP			
POTATOES, MAINCROP										OCT	NOV	DEC
RASPBERRIES							JUL	AUG				
RHUBARB					MAY	JUN	JUL					
SPINACH					MAY	JUN	JUL	AUG	SEP	OCT		
STRAWBERRIES						JUN	JUL	AUG				
SQUASH									SEP	OCT		
SWEETCORN								AUG	SEP	OCT		

In step 17 we looked at the benefits of eating fresh local produce. Here you can find what fruit and vegetables are in season around the year. This is so that if you aren't able to get to a farmers' market. You can still try to buy produce that is in season from your local supermarket.

The labels on fresh produce will tell you where it was grown or reared anyway (unless it says "produce o more than one country"), but if it's in season in your part of the world, there's a higher chance of it being grown locally too.

Step 18 - Eat only seasonal foods for a week

You may find that the foods that are in season are better suited to the current climate and easy to incorporate into your meal plan anyway.
.
Make a meal plan for the week using mainly foods in season and the shop for it.

"Eat organic, local and seasonal, it's how our ancestors lived so long"

Leah Salmon

110

To make this step a success, this week I am committed to:

_____

_____

_____

_____

_____

_____

_____

_____

_____

_____

By the end of this week I hope to:

_____

_____

_____

_____

_____

Step 19 – Mix It Up A Bit

It's been found that by the time a man is in his late 20's, he only knows how to make 3 different meals and people in general will eat the same 4 or 5 meals most of the time. This is kind of boring don't you think? Considering there are 300 varieties of fruit, 100's of vegetables, grains, nuts, seeds, seaweeds, herb, spices, meats and fishes to choose from.

Religious and conscious beliefs may limit the animals you eat, which is quite understandable, but there is a world of other culinary treats available to you. Try to eat at different restaurants (ones recommended to you are best and feel free to call ahead to find out where they source their ingredients and if they can cater fro your needs), buy cook books from different countries, try meals and foods from your own country that you've never tried before.

Once every few months, treat yourself to the most expensive, fruits, nuts, fishes, ingredients and seasonings to discover how great (or sometimes terrible) they taste. Allowing a wide array of foods into your diet can also increase the range of nutrients, especially trace elements you get.

If you have children, it can be beneficial for them to get a wider range of nutrients from different foods and allows them to find their favourite foods from a bigger spectrum, instead of just eating what their parents are used to making. It's also a life experience for you all to at least sample foods, flavours and textures from around the global.

Using the following table, find and taste the foods listed and find some of your own you'd like to try too. If there are some you like but haven't had in a while, add them to the menu soon.

New Food	Tired it and loved it	Tried it, didn't like it	Would like to try it
Romanesco			
Breadfruit			
Cherimoya (Custard Apple)			
Jack Fruit			
Dragon Fruit			
Tamarind			
Okra			
Water Chestnuts			
Young Jelly Coconuts			
Nori			
Arame			
Amaranth			
Tahini			

Step 19 - Once a day for the next week, eat something you've never tried before

---

To make this step a success, this week I am committed to:

_____

_____

_____

_____

_____

_____

_____

_____

By the end of this week I hope to:

_____

_____

_____

_____

Step 20 – Rawsome

I've been a lover and support of the health benefits of raw live fresh foods for a number of years now after being introduced to the topic by The Raw Food Coach Karen Knowler and Jingee & Storm Talifero from The Garden Diet.

To get the full scoop on the joys of raw foods, plus 100 delicious recipes and meal plans, grab yourself a copy of my book "Leah's Raw Food Feast from my site www.TheNaturallyYouCoach.com.

But in short, just some of the benefits of including more fresh live raw foods to your life are:

Raw foods:
Taste great
Are a good source of water
Are a great source of fibre
Can be very healing to the body
Aren't addictive like many cooked foods
Provide vitamins, minerals and nutrients in their natural form
Have active enzymes, which are essential to vibrant health
Satisfy your hunger without making you feel stuffed or heavy
Can take very little time to prepare
Taste great (did I mention that already!!!)

There is a myth that accompanies talk of raw food, that say to get the true benefits you HAVE TO go 100% raw long term. This is NOT A FACT.

Some people go fully raw and do amazing well, while others spend years raw then go back to eating other foods due to nutritional deficiencies or simply missing other wholesome cooked foods.

What I have found is that adding more nutrient rich raw foods to your life and diet never ceases to benefit your health.

To give you a taste of the joys of raw food, here are a few of my favourite recipes to get your raw taste buds going

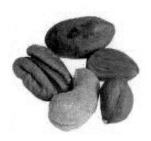

Pecan Nut and Date Milk
Even though almond milk is most popular, I quite like the richness of pecans, which are a good source of fibre.

Ingredients
1 cup (150g) of pecans
3 cups of pure water
4-5 soft dates, pitted

Directions: Soak the nuts overnight in the water. In the morning (or about 6 hours later), drain the nuts and blend them in 3 cups of fresh water until they are completely broken down, this could take about 1-2 minutes stopping the machine every 30 seconds or so, unless you are using a very powerful blender (Vitamix, Blentec etc).

Once it's all blended, strain the milk, pour the milk back into the blender with the dates and blend again for another 30 seconds and enjoy.

To make a thicker richer smoothie, blend in a banana or some raw chocolate or carob powder for a chocolate milkshake.

Succulent Broccoli and Ginger Salad
The thought of raw broccoli may not seem very appealing at first, but this is definitely worth a try.

Ingredients
1 head of broccoli
½ a inch of fresh ginger
¼ cup of Extra Virgin Olive Oil
A pinch of salt and a squeeze of lemon juice

Directions: Wash and chop the broccoli finely. Mince the ginger by finely chopping or pressing it through a garlic press. Stir the ginger into the broccoli along with the olive oil, salt and lemon juice. Massaging everything into the broccoli will help it really absorb the flavours.

Once it's well mixed, you can either leave it in the airing cupboard overnight or put it in a dehydrator for about 2 hours. This will help soften the broccoli slightly so it will absorb the flavours.

This can be served on a green leaf salad, topped with chopped tomatoes or avocados or as a side to any meal. Enjoy!

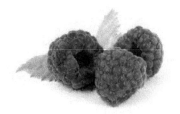

Pink ice Cream
This creamy sorbet has all the taste and texture of diary ice cream with out the sugar or mucus filled pasteurised cows milk

Ingredients
200g frozen raspberries
2 bananas peeled, chopped and frozen until solid
1 cup of fresh orange juice

Directions
Simply place everything into a blender and blend until smooth and creamy. It' best made in a high speed blender or a smoothie maker with a tamper to push the frozen banana safely down into the blades (please only use a tamper that comes with your blender). In the absence of a high speed blender, use a food processor instead.

One of the most convincing arguments for including more raw foods into your diet is that many raw foods retain more nutrients.

Here are just 2 examples of the difference between raw and cooked foods.

		Calcium	Vit C	Iron
	Raw	33mg	5.9mg	0.30mg
	Cooked	30mg	3.6mg	0.34mg
Carrots	Based on 100g of raw and 100g of cooked & drained carrots			

		Calcium	Vit C	Potassium
Broccoli	**Raw**	47mg	89.2mg	316mg
	Cooked	40mg	64mg	297mg
	Based on 100g of raw and 100g of cooked, drained broccoli			

These figures are taken from the United States Department Of Agriculture's Nutrient Data Laboratory (www.nal.usda.gov/fnic/foodcomp/search/index.html)

There are examples of vegetables whose vitamin and mineral levels increase with low temperature cooking on this website also, however we know that all the enzymes and phytonutrients would be destroyed once cooked

Step 20 - Make 50% or more of your food raw a day this week.

You can do this by having a raw breakfast of vegetables, fruits, nuts and soaked grains and then a salad or other raw food for half of your lunch and dinner.

To make this step a success, this week I am committed to:

_____

_____

_____

_____

_____

_____

_____

_____

_____

_____

By the end of this week I hope to:

_____

_____

_____

_____

_____

Step 21 – Get Your Greens

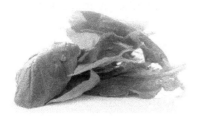

Having spent my teens as a "Junk Food vegetarian", whose diet was mainly processed carbs or soya meat replacements, when I started adding whole colourful foods to my plate it was a big step.

Most of my foods was brown (soya burgers, soya mince, chocolate), white (pasta, rice, chips) or yellow and red (cheese and pizza).

So the juicy red tomatos, bell peppers, watermelons and radishes, yellow bananas and lemons and orange carrots, pumpkins and mangos provided me with more colour and the nutrients associated with those natural colours.

But the biggest jump was in the green foods, which made up a lot of my diet and were the least appetising to look at to begin with too (I bet you can relate).

I was just as squeamish about drinking 'green goop' as most of the people I work with today.

But I'm glad I got over this initial hurdle, as green foods come in so many shapes and sizes and give you a whole host of health boosting nutrients.

Top Five Benefits of Green Foods

1. They are nutrient powerhouses and even contain chlorophyll, which captures the sun's energy in a form we can ingest.
2. Many of them are high in an easy to use fibre to help digestion, cleansing, absorption and make them more filling, especially in their raw or lightly cooked state.
3. They are high in lutein which prevents visual degeneration
4. They are so versatile that they can be easily added to salads, stews, smoothies, juices and many other foods
5. There are always some type of greens in season all year round, so they are never going to be too expensive or too hard to find locally and organically

To get you in the swing of things, here are some simple ways of adding more greens to your diet.

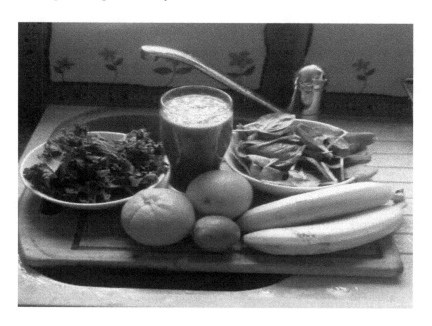

Green smoothie recipes
You'll need:

| A big handful of spinach | 1 cup of orange juice |
| 2 bananas | 1 cup of water |

Or

| The flesh of 1 large mango | 1 cup of water |
| 2 apple | 1 handful of kale |

Put all ingredients for either recipe in a blender and blend until smooth.

Do you find salads boring? Firstly a few splashes of homemade or natural salad dressing can spruce it up and maybe you need to change the green leaves you're using! Here are some you can choose from:

Romaine Lettuce	Parsley	Sorrel
Rocket	Spinach	Sunflower greens
Lambs Lettuce	Spring greens	Alfalfa Sprouts
Water Cress	Dandelion greens	Endive
Coriander	Basil	Swiss Chard
Kale	Parsley	Sorrell

Step 21 – Have greens twice a day for a week.

You can do this by having a green smoothie with or for your breakfast every morning and have a big green salad with or as one of your meals every day.

To make this step a success, this week I am committed to:

_____

_____

_____

_____

_____

_____

_____

_____

_____

_____

_____

By the end of this week I hope to:

_____

_____

_____

_____

_____

Step 22 – Get It Organic

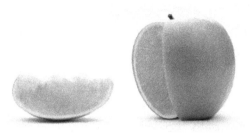

"Confused, so you should be, if they can mix animals DNA into vegetables to get a better product, are you eating a vegetable, an animal or a genetic mutation, anyone care for an apple orange?"

Even though many people try and deny the benefits of organic foods, recent studies have shown that it IS in fact better for you than conventionally farmed produce or reared meats, poultry and eggs.

Amongst the many arguments given to include more organic food into your diet, here are the top 3 reasons I choose organic over conventionally farmed foods as much as I possible can, especially for our children.

Taste – This may be different for different people, but personally, the difference in taste between organic and non organic foods to me is remarkable, especially sweetcorn, apples, sweet potatoes, carrots, broccoli, mushrooms, most types of tomatoes and bananas. Other foods can taste as good whether they are organic or not, but the above seem to have, not only more flavour, but they look and smell fresher and more nutritious too.

Nutrients – A £12million 4 year study led by Newcastle University, UK, found that organically grown fruits, vegetables and milk from organically reared cattle were more nutritious than the conventionally grown and reared produce. Milk from the organic cows had 30% more antioxidants and organic wheat, tomatoes, potatoes, cabbage, onions were found to contain 40% more nutrients than normal produce.

Safety – There are over 300 chemical fertilisers and pesticides that are used on conventionally farmed food, most of which are sprayed directly onto the skins. So foods with edible skins like apples, grapes, tomatoes, pears, berries etc. are still going to have residues of these chemicals on them when they reach my kitchen.

There are products available like Veggie Wash and natural solutions like apple cider vinegar, that you can use to clean the skin of fruits and vegetable to get rid of these chemicals, but a certain amount will penetrate the skins and become a part of the foods.

To me the thought of this, and the fact that the safety to humans when exposed to the cocktail of chemicals hasn't been researched well enough at all, is enough to convince me that the extra cost is worth it.

What can I do if I can afford to only eat organic foods?
As organic foods typically cost more than conventionally farmed foods (but not always), there is a handy list produced by the Environmental Working Group (EWG) called "The Dirty Dozen and Clean Fifteen".

Ever year this organisation tests the level of pesticides, herbicides and chemical residues on and in 50 different fruits and vegetables and condense their findings into a list of the "Dirty Dozen", which are the 12 foods which are best bought organic as they have the most residues on and in them and the "Clean Fifteen" which are the 15 foods that are safer to buy commercially grown as they typically have the least. You can find them at www.ewg.org/foodnews, where you can download the free guide for the current year.

There are also some companies in the UK that deliver boxes of organic food to your door each week to make it more convenient for you to add more. They sell not just fruit and vegetables, but also meats, fish, poultry, eggs, breads, pastries and most cupboard and fridge foods. Able & Cole and Riverford Organic are my 2 favourites, but I know there are some other great ones.

You can also see if there's a local Food Co Op operating in your area. This is when a group of people get together and buy organic or healthy foods in bulk and then split the cost between them to make it cheaper.

In recent years there have been several documentaries showing the effects of genetically modified foods on human health and the benefits of eating more organic food, which include:

Forks Over Knives
Food Inc
Food Matter
Hungry For Change
The Future Of Food
Ingredients

If you've watched any others that you can recommend, please let me know so I can add them to future revisions of this book.

Step 22 – Up your organic for a week

You can do this by choosing 5 of your regular foods and getting them organic for a week or you can prepare one organic meal a day for a week. If you already eat a lot of organic and want to go fully organic this week, go for it!!!

To make this step a success, this week I am committed to:

_____

_____

_____

_____

_____

_____

By the end of this week I hope to:

_____

_____

_____

_____

Step 23 – Eat Right For Your Type

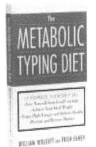 Did you know that there's not one diet that suits every single person on the planet?

Did you know that we all have a unique requirement for nutrients to experience optimum health?

Have you heard of a process called Metabolic Typing that focuses on the biochemical individuality of a person to determine what balance of nutrients works best for them?

Hippocrates once said "It is more important to know what type of patient has a disease, than to know what type of disease a patient has", which sums up what Metabolic Typing is.

It's about eating right for your body type, finding out how your body works and starting to build your health, through nutrition, from there.

You've probably noticed that there are hundreds of books on diet & nutrition around these days. That being the case, why is it then, in a time when we are more health, diet and exercise conscious than ever, that cancer, heart disease and obesity are increasing every year?

Why do some people lose weight on a high protein diet or high carb diet, but the same diet will make someone else put on weight?

And the million dollar question

"How can someone eat the best organic foods, take the finest nutritional supplements that money can buy, get plenty of rest, exercise regularly . . . And Still Not Feel Well ?

Metabolic Typing provides an answer

Your metabolic type is the *inherited patterns* of biochemical and neurological *strengths and weaknesses* that make up your metabolic individuality.

So like no two snowflakes are the same – on an individual level, we are all as unique as our fingerprints. There's an infinite diversity in metabolic individuality from our physical structure, psychological make-up, to the size and position of our internal organs and glands - everyone has inherited specific requirements for nutrition....

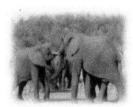 ....just like lions rarely eat leaves and elephants don't eat meat!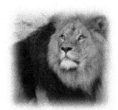

The concept of Metabolic Typing or MT isn't new, for thousands of years, humans have traveled and migrated to different parts of the planet and while there they had to adapt to their new environment.

So the forces of evolution assured human survival on local foods and ancestral diets were established all over the world.

In 1930 a man by the name of Dr Weston Price, originally a dentist, wanted to find out why so many Americans suffered with tooth decay, gum disease and crowded teeth, when undeveloped regions of the world had no such problems.

So he visited 14 of these ancestral tribes in a bid to find out more.

Amongst his findings were that the Masai in Africa lived on a diet of meat, milk, blood extracted from cattle and had extraordinary physical and mental development.

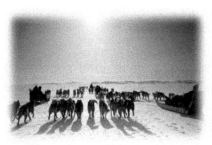 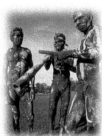

Eskimos ate a diet with large quantities of meat and fat like caribou, kelp, salmon, moose, seal and whale blubber, yet cardiovascular disease was virtually unknown. The Aboriginals survived on insects, grubs, berries, kangaroo and wallaby meat and had great strength and fitness levels and the Indians of South America exist largely on a vegetable diet with virtually no disease. In general he found that all their diets had:

- No refined of devitalized foods
- Sweets, even natural sugars were used very rarely
- Most foods were eaten raw or very slightly cooked
- All foods were organic, seasonal and eaten freely
- They enjoyed regular physical exercise and periods of foods abstinence
- Adequate unpolluted fresh air
- And health giving sunlight

They did suffer from headaches, colds, wounds, burns and accidents, but they had NO cavities, degenerative diseases or emotional problems like depression.

Their diets were tremendously varied. When these people left their native diets and adopted modern eating habits (processed carbs, racid fats etc), they fell prey to the same degenerative diseases that plague modern society.

Then you get to the supposedly developed countries like North America, the United Kingdom and Australia where the populations are now essentially *'genetic mosaics',* with no clear-cut ethnic or genetic heritage, no genetically determined diet, yet plenty of disease.

So what is disease? Diseases *are* actually the outward expressions of internal imbalances, so diseases aren't the problems that need treatment. Once you can metabolise your food and turn it fully into energy, you can correct imbalances and your body can heal itself.

Two people with the same disease may have opposite imbalances and different metabolic types. You can have two people with high blood pressure, one may be a carnivore and the other a vegetarian. So to treat all people nutritionally the same for each disease won't work.

You still have the freedom to follow your chosen diet, but when you know your type, you can adjust it to suit you. Two people can be vegetarians and ones a protein type, while the other is a carb type and as long as they adapt the vegetarian food to their needs they can both thrive.

Some myths that surround nutrition

A vegetarian or low fat/low protein, high complex carbohydrate diet is good for you – well if it's wrong for your Metabolic Type, it can worsen your condition. The Atkins / South Beach / Zone / Paleo / Primal / Raw Food diet is the ideal diet for everyone – well as you may have gathered so far, there is no such thing as a universally healthy diet that is right for all people.

To lose weight, simply reduce calories, exercise and eat a well-balanced diet – the reality is that fat doesn't make you fat. Protein doesn't make you fat. Carbs don't make you fat. Calories don't even make you fat . . . but an inefficient metabolism does.

Different Metabolic Types require
- Different _kinds_ of foods
- Different _balances_ of nutrients
- Different _ratios_ of protein/fat/carbohydrate
- Some metabolic types will do well on a largely vegetarian diet like the east Indians and some will thrive on a carnivores diet like the Eskimos

There are 6 main metabolic types

Autonomic Types	Oxidative Types	Generally referred to as
Parasympathetic	Fast oxidiser	"Protein Types"
Sympathetic	Slow oxidiser	"Carbohydrate Types"
Balanced	Mixed oxidiser	"Mixed Types"

No one can really say how it will affect you, but as a Metabolic Typing Advisor for the past 6 years, the main advantages my clients have reported are:

Increased Sustainable Energy – Not having a sluggish feeling after eating and not waking up tired and going to bed tired. Clients eating whole foods right for their Metabolic Type finally have the energy they never had before to complete tasks without effort, exercise more, think more clearly and live a more fulfilling life.

Weight Normalisation – When clients ask for a Metabolic Typing program to help them lose weight, I always tell them that first you find your health, then weight loss will follow. However, those who are looking to gain weight also benefit from this program. The term weight normalisation is most appropriate because crash dieting or rapid weight loss or weight gain programs can cause a yo-yo effect on weight where you'll lose 10lbs one week and gain 20lbs the next. Metabolic Typing helps you to steadily reach the weight that is best for you, if you want to lose or gain weight, this can also be done steadily and in tune with your body.

Freedom From Food Cravings - There are so many people around who have food cravings that are seriously impacting their health, but many of them don't realise this until they try and take away the food they crave. For example, someone may deny having a craving for coffee and caffeine products, but when they stop their morning, mid morning and after lunch coffee by dinner time they complain of headaches, anxiety, irritability and strong cravings for coffee and sweets.

Those that are more aware of their cravings, don't know how to control them so simply give in to them constantly.

One very important thing to remember is that, oftentimes, when you crave something it's because your body is lacking in a particular nutrient so it pushes you to seek out that nutrient. Because junks foods are typical comfort foods too, we tend to go to these first before seeking out the natural alternative.

So when our body is lacking fats for example, many of us head for chips, pizza or greasy fried foods instead of an avocado, nuts and seeds or meat and oily fish. When your diet is comprised of whole foods that provide you with nutrients that are right for you, your physical cravings will go leaving you with just your cravings that have psychological roots and with naturally you coaching, these can be overcome too.

Reversal and prevention of disease and illness – It is not uncommon to hear of people's digestive problems, skin conditions, constant headaches, aches and pains clearing up after some time on a Metabolic Typing diet, as the body finally has the fuel and energy to balance and heal things that have been going wrong. But in the words of the great Dr Malachi Z York, don't believe me, check it out for yourself.

135

Step 23 – Discover your Metabolic Type and eat according to it for a week

You can find free online tests or buy the book "Metabolic Typing Diet" by William Wolcott or "How To Eat Move & Be Healthy" by Paul Chek which both have basic tests in them to find out your Metabolic Type.

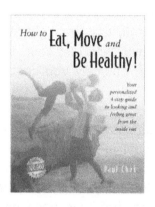 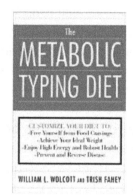

Or you can visit www.thenaturallyyoucoach.com , click on coaching and look at The Naturally You Personalised Diet & Life Plan, for an advanced test and additional support. Once you've used any of the above to discover your Metabolic Type, eat according to the recommendations you're given for a week at least and see how you feel.

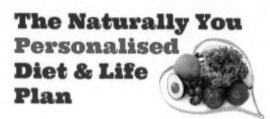

To make this step a success, this week I am committed to:

_____

_____

_____

_____

_____

_____

_____

_____

_____

_____

By the end of this week I hope to:

_____

_____

_____

_____

_____

_____

_____

Step 24 – Sprout It

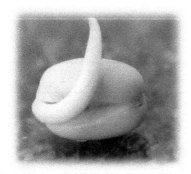

Super sprouts to the rescue

Nuts, grains, beans and seeds all become more nutritious when they are soaked before cooking. This is because in their dry state, they contain enzyme inhibitors which make them indigestible and in a dormant state.

This is so that while in nature, until they find the right conditions for growth they won't rot. Whether you plant them in the ground and water them or soak them in water overnight, once exposed to enough moisture for a certain amount of time, nutrients in them become activated and available, either to make a healthier more digestible food to eat or to give it nutrients and energy to grow into a new plant in the ground.

Once soaked, live enzymes are also formed, which make them an energy boosting food and further help our bodies to digest them.

As the name suggests, you will see a sprout and eventually a green shoot begin growing from what your sprouting, which if left to continue could grow into a plant of that food.

Sprouts are famous for their energy and protein content so they are great for those who are lacking protein or energy while adding more raw food to their diet.

They are also useful for vegetarians, vegans and raw vegans who are found to be protein metabolic types.

Want to grow your own super healthy sprouts? It's so simple and here's how you do it.

How to sprout your own Alfalfa seeds

For me these are one of the easiest seeds to sprout and they produce a great yield, about 3 tbsp of seeds can make 3 cups of sprouts. If you have a sprouting tray or machine it should come with instructions, this method is for beginners and requires just a glass jar.

You'll need:

A large glass jar that you can fit your hand into
An elastic band
A piece of muslin, cheesecloth, some type of clean material with fine holes in it or some clean unused tights
3 tablespoons of alfalfa seeds (widely available online or in health food stores)

Directions

1. Half fill the jar with clean water and pour in the seeds.
2. Place the muslin or tights over the top of the jar and secure with the elastic band.
3. Leave the seeds to soak overnight on your kitchen counter, somewhere not too hot or too cold, then the next day, pour out the water, rinse with fresh water, drain very well through the tights or muslin, then leave the soaked seeds to sprout for about 8 hours. Make sure the seeds are drained well and aren't sitting in a puddle of water as they won't sprout as well.
4. After about 8 hours or at least twice a day, maybe once in the morning, then the early evening, rinse, drain well and leave the seeds to sprout.

5. After about 3 - 5 days, the alfalfa sprouts will have fully sprouted, meaning first a white shoot, then small green leaves will grow from the seeds. Now they are ready to eat and enjoy. The warmer the environment the quicker they will sprout.
6. They will keep on growing and growing and growing until they eventually start to rot, so once they are ready to eat (at about 1cm long) put them in the fridge to slow down their growth and then eat them within 3 days.

Other seeds and grains you can try and sprout (times may vary)

Chickpeas	Mung Beans	Sunflower Seeds
Red or Green lentils	Quiona	Pumpkin Seeds
Fenugreek	Red Clover	broccoli seed
Aduki Beans	Radish	

Soaking Before Cooking
Even though you can eat many grains, legumes and seeds raw once soaked and sprouted, it's also a very good idea to soak them before cooking them too. Some of the nutrients activated in the soaking process aren't easily harmed by heat and will make your cooked food more nutritious and easy to digest too.

Rice, beans, lentils, oats, quinoa and other grains can all be soaked over night and drained before cooking, which also helps to reduce cooking time

Nuts & Seeds For Smoothies or Nut Milks
Soaking the raw nuts and seeds you want to make smoothies from overnight, will also make them more nutritious and easy to digest, giving you more nutrients from them once made.

WARNING!!!

Make sure you soak your Kidney beans before cooking them, but make sure you don't eat them as raw sprouts as they aren't safe to eat until cooked.

How To Eat Sprouts

Sprouts go well in salads, a topping for soups, in sandwiches, smoothies, juices and anywhere you would normally use salad greens.

"Soak and sprout grains, nuts and seeds to give your body the nutrients it needs"

Leah Salmon

Step 24 – Eat sprouts twice a day for a week
You can put a few spoons on your lunch and dinner plates or blend them into your green smoothies or even vegetable juices.

To make this step a success, this week I am committed to:

_____

_____

_____

_____

_____

_____

_____

_____

_____

_____

By the end of this week I hope to:

_____

_____

_____

_____

_____

Step 25 – Herbs, Spices & Salt

One of the things that differentiate a good cook from someone who just makes food, is their ability to use seasonings and cooking techniques to change the way something tastes. They can make carrots come alive, rice taste divine, chicken taste juicy and succulent and a salad taste incredible.

There was once a time when the use of natural herbs, spices and salts were used for this, but nowadays, there are stacks of readymade seasonings on supermarket shelves that have taken that job completely out of our hands.

This can be a really convenient way to season your food, but the downside is that a great deal of readymade seasonings contain chemicals like the dreaded MSG we spoke about in Step 12, sugar, refined salt and sometimes colourings and preservatives. Using fresh or dried herbs, spices and natural salts to season your food, can prevent you from taking in these chemicals on a regular basis and naturally enhance the flavour and nutritional content of your foods too.

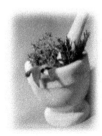

Herbs
These can be added to your food the same way you would normally add seasonings, though fresh herbs are best added 5 minutes before the end so their flavour remains strong in the food when served.

I have found that you can also freeze fresh herbs that you are going to cook with, but they don't last as long as if dried.

Here are some herbs you can commonly get fresh or dried, that you can try in your cooking:

Basil	Sage	Thyme
Coriander	Lemongrass	Parsley
Mustard	Mint	Bay Leaves
Chives	Fennel	Rosemary
Oregano	Curry leaves	Dill

Spices

My mother comes from Grenada, which is known as the Island Of Spice, so I grew up eating cornmeal porridge every Saturday and sometimes Sunday mornings (although Sunday's breakfast was normally reserved for kippers). My mum would always season it with nutmeg grated from the actual nutmeg bulbs and a whole stick of cinnamon. I would always try and fish out the cinnamon stick so I could suck the porridge through it, it tasted sweet, pungent and delicious. Here are some more natural spices you can use to season your sweet or savoury dishes:

Cloves	Vanilla beans	Cayenne
Ginger	Pimento	Smoked Paprika
Star Anise	Cumin	Saffron

A word on Salt

A diet too high in highly processed table salt isn't good for your health as you may have heard, however there are some very nutritious salts that are a health giving addition to your meals. So opt for these over table salt:

Celtic Sea Salt	Herbamere Salt
Himalayan Crystal Salt	Grey Sea Salt

144

Step 25 – Only use herbs, spices and natural salts to season your food this week. If you find a herb or spice blend, be sure to check the ingredients first.

To make this step a success, this week I am committed to:

_____

_____

_____

_____

_____

_____

_____

_____

By the end of this week I hope to:

_____

_____

_____

_____

Step 26 – Know Your Oils

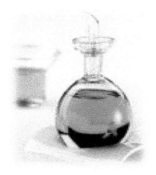 If I had released this book a few years ago, I'd have to spend a few paragraphs convincing you all that fat doesn't actually make you fat, we need good fats in our diet and that too little fat for anyone, even those who do better on lower fat diets, can be detrimental to your health.

So in this step, we're going to get straight to the stuff you really need to know about fats and oils.

What's so Essential about Essential Fatty Acids?
In short, our body can't make essential fatty acids the way that it can make saturated fats, so we have to get them from our foods. Once our bodies have a sufficient supply of essential fatty acids, it can manufacture other essential nutrients for health like prostaglandin, which are essential hormone like substances in the body.

Are saturated fats and cholesterol the absolute enemy?
Both of these are found in your body naturally. Your body actually needs cholesterol to produce steroids and saturated fats are used to provide a source of energy, help build cell membrane, carry fat soluble vitamins and help the conversion of carotene to vitamin A for mineral absorption and other vital processes.

Saturated fats from organic, natural vegetable and animal sources are part of a health giving diet. It's the overproduction or intake of these substances in the wrong body types that cause a problem.

146

Protein metabolic types can handle and thrive on high levels of fats, which in them won't lead to diseases normally associated with high saturated fat diets. Whereas a carbohydrate type can't handle fats as well and is likely to develop the conditions commonly associated with high fat diets, as well as just feeling tired, heavy and low on energy.

So to determine how much is best for you, you'd first need to find out your metabolic type then fine-tune your diet to find the levels that are suited to you personally (see Step 23).

So no, saturated fats and cholesterol aren't the enemy, you just need to eat wholesome clean sources of them and find the level that's right for your body type.

What's really so bad about white oils?

The process of turning seeds and nuts into the clear, colourless, odourless, tasteless liquids you see on the supermarket shelves, goes a little something like this. Bear in mind that the seeds and nuts in their original raw state contain oil that is highly nutritious and health giving:

1. Firstly seeds are mechanically cleaned.
2. Then the seeds are either cooked and the oil is mechanically pressed out, under processes which produce high levels of heat, or they are flaked and a solvent (like hexane found in gasoline, yes, you read it correctly, the same stuff you put in your car) is used to extract the oil from the seed.
3. The oil is then degummed to remove fibre and lecithin, which is then isolated and sold as a supplement.
4. The degummed oil will then be refined using something like caustic soda, which is strong enough to clean your drains.

5. The resulting red or yellow oil is now bleached to remove the colour pigments chlorophyll and beta carotene, as well as natural aromatic substances, which all help to increase the shelf life of the oil.
6. Now to further remove any remaining unpleasant odours and tastes that have resulted from the previous processing steps (that weren't there in the natural oils) the oil is deodorised.
7. The resulting oil is now ready to hit the shelves for us to consume at ridiculously high levels every year.

Did you know that children in the UK who eat just one packet of crisps a day (and there are some eating 2, 3 or even 15) are drinking 5 litres of rancid oil a year!!!

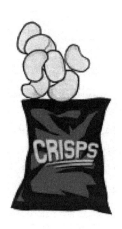

Each of the stages listed above subjects the oils to the 3 things that cause them to go rancid

Heat – *Light* – *Oxygen*

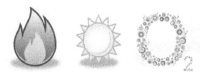

Each stage removes more and more vitamins, minerals, fibre, flavour, fatty acids and natural aroma. Leaving us with a clear tasteless, odourless, nutrient dead, good for little liquid.

So what's the alternative?
There are a number of alternatives to eating these oils that will positively impact your health and vitality.

Oils to cook with
Most oils become rancid on exposure to heat, especially vegetable oils. The only oils that are shown to be more stable when heated and therefore better to cook with are *Coconut oil, Palm oil, Ghee, real butter and to a lesser degree Extra Virgin Olive oil.*

Oils to add to food once cooked
These are oils that are ok to be stored at room temperature in a dark cool place, but not great to heat to high temperatures, so adding them to your food once it's cooked can still add flavour and texture to your meals: *Olive Oil & Sesame Oil*

Nutritional Oils Which Should Be Kept Refrigerated
These oils are most unstable at high temperatures and to retain their full potency, they should be kept away from heat, light and oxygen as much as possible. They can still be added to food once it's cooked and on your plate. Remember, before oils leave the seeds or nuts, they are encased in the shell of the seed or nut and protected from these elements naturally: *Hemp Oil, Flaxseed Oil and Fermented Cod Liver Oil*

Ways To Add Nutritional Oils To Your Diet

- Warm very slightly and infuse with garlic or herbs and use as a dip for homemade or good quality bread
- Stir into porridges or muesli
- Stir into soups
- Blend into a smoothie or juice
- Stir into fruit puree or yoghurt
- Use to make mayonnaise, humus or pesto

Step 26 – Use oils according to the points above and include a nutritional oil to your life for a week

---

West Indian, African and Asian markets are good places to find these oils as many of them are from these parts of the world.

To make this step a success, this week I am committed to:

_____

_____

_____

_____

_____

_____

_____

_____

_____

_____

By the end of this week I hope to:

_____

_____

_____

_____

_____

Step 27 – Be Snack Savvy

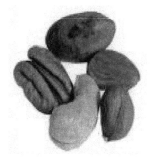

Do we need to snack?

This all depends on what type of person you are, your body type and nutritional needs. If you have very well balanced and fulfilling meals and plenty of water, you'll have more stable blood sugar levels and will typically be able to do without snacks.

However, there are some people who 'live to eat' and so do well when they snack between meals, if they don't snack, they get low blood sugar symptoms, can't functional optimally and without anything planned, they may resort to junk food and sweets to tide them over.

There are others who 'eat to live'; they are quite disinterested in food, don't mind if they skip a meal and rarely if ever need to snack between meals. If this is you, unless you are following a particular program with a professional, there is no need to force yourself to eat, just listen to your body.

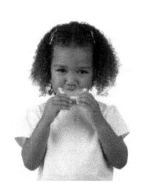

Children's Snacks

I had such a hard time working out whether or not to let my children snack, when they should snack and what to snack on. In short though, children are typically active and burn energy quickly, which needs to be replaced regularly.

If you are able to give your children 3 substantial meals a day with plenty of water in between, they may not actually need snacks, but always have healthy snacks to hand if your children do need more between meals. The balancing act comes in when you work out how many snacks is enough to fulfil them between meals, without it interfering with their main meals. I talk much more about how to feed children a healthy diet in my book on healthy eating for children coming soon.

When To Snack

For some people, having set snack times in the day, keeps them from just grazing (constantly picking at food). It can be helpful to set times to snack if you are changing your eating habits, starting a new program or you're used to comfort eating, just until you're comfortable with everything. But typically, there is no real need to set times to snack and as long as you only have wholesome foods around that you only eat when you are truly hungry and not just bored or restless.

What to snack on - Healthy snack Choices

Small portions of left overs or main meals
Raw vegetable sticks with humus or nut/seed butters
Humus on raw crackers or breads
Rye or spelt bread & avocado slices
Raw nuts and seeds
Nut or seed smoothies
Chicken legs or boiled eggs
Cherry tomatoes, baby plum tomatoes or sugar snap peas
Vegetable juices
Green smoothies
Fresh fruit or vegetable salads
Tuna or chicken salad
Steamed broccoli & green beans with olive oil & sea salt

Step 27 – Replace unhealthy snacks with whole food healthy alternatives for a week

Planning what snacks you'll have with you will stop the biggest source of unhealthy snacking for many of us which is impulse snack buying when you're out and of course, if you buy unhealthy snacks in your groceries that are in your home, get them out of your home or environment for this week

To make this step a success, this week I am committed to:

_____

_____

_____

_____

_____

_____

By the end of this week I hope to:

_____

_____

_____

Step 28 – Fail To Plan, Plan To Fail

Once you are in the swing of things in your new healthier lifestyle, things are likely to just flow with little or no planning, You'll know which meals work best for you, you'll know recipes off by heart, your fridge and cupboards will be well stocked with only the foods that work well for you and you'll know exactly what to do with them.

If you have already reached that place in your life, then this section may not be too important to you, but if you are just getting into a healthy lifestyle, these pointers could help steer you in the right direction.

Even if you aren't one for sticking to a plan, doing some brief planning initially can really help in the long run. It can be something you look back on if you lose focus or come off track along the way.

What is there to plan???
This is actually a good question because you may not realise what to plan, much less the benefit of planning it.

The answer is, as much as you can.

So once you've decided what you want to achieve with your health, food, lifestyle or environment, write it down, followed by what it will take to achieve it. Keep the information in the plan simple but detailed enough to make it comprehensive and easy to follow.

Here's an example

Becoming Naturally You

Goal	Steps Needed
Cut out MSG from my diet	1. Find all the foods I have/use with MSG in them 2. Find alternatives for them & don't buy them again
Drink at least 6 glasses of water daily	1. Get rid of the juice and sodas I have in the house 2. Buy a few glass 1 litre bottles and fill one a day with water and pinch of salt. Keep one next to my bed, one on my desk at work and in the living room 5. Set alarm on my phone every 2 hours from 9am – 7pm to remind me to drink
Go raw one day a week	1. Work out what I want to eat during that day, get the recipes and buy all the ingredients 2 days before 2. Spend 1hour the night before soaking, sprouting, marinating or dehydrating what I'll need and go to bed early. 3. Have a brilliant day on raw foods!!!
Stop eating rice, bread & pasta	1. Write a meal plan for the week that doesn't include them, but is really yummy 2. Do shopping for the week to get all the ingredients I need plus some snacks or special foods I like 3. Throw out or give away all the rice, bread and pasta I have, stick to the meal plan and treat myself with the special foods if I get grumpy.

156

Carrying out this quick brainstorm before you pursue your goal can save you time by not having to keep stopping along the way to work things out. It can save you money, as you've already planned what to buy and are less likely to impulse buy on a whim.

It also allows you to be creative and adventurous yet practical. You can really work out what you'd love to do, be and achieve and take the time to work out exactly what you can realistically do to achieve it.

So if you've always wanted to try a vegan or raw vegan diet for example, you can plan what it would take to do it for maybe 3-5 days, the recipes and different foods you'd like to try, where to get the recipes and foods from and all of a sudden, what seemed like a far off dream, can quickly become a very achievable reality. You can even find a raw or vegan restaurant to treat yourself too.

Step 28 – Think of a food goal you have at the moment and make a plan to achieve it this week

You can use a table like the one in the examples above to simply plan what you need to do.

Choose a goal that is fairly challenging and out of your comfort zone, but that will have a big impact on your life and health

---

To make this step a success, this week I am committed to:

_____

_____

_____

_____

_____

_____

_____

_____

_____

_____

_____

By the end of this week I hope to:

_____

_____

_____

_____

_____

Step 29 – Know How To Work A Budget

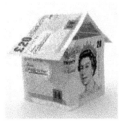 One of the common misconceptions that people have about eating a more wholesome diet is that it costs the earth. Well if you use several different superfoods, buy loads of raw snack bars and raw chocolate, take 5 different natural supplements a day and eat all organic food, then yes it'll cost a lot.

It all depends how far you want to take it. There are ways to eat more simple, wholesome and cost effective foods on a budget. With a house full of 5 children who all eat a predominantly wholefood diet, I have "healthy eating on a budget" down to a fine art, believe me it's very possible.

Planning - If you know what you want to make, only buy the things you need, without impulse buying things you don't end up using which wastes money.

Cook, Freeze or dry bargains - If you see fresh foods on sale, buy loads of them and dehydrate, freeze or cook meals with them that you freeze, so you have them in stock. Obviously make sure they are still within the use by date and look and smell fresh.

Make It yourself - Buying the ingredients for your own sandwiches, soups and meals can be cheaper than buying readymade stuff everyday for lunch, Buy bags of fruit instead of buying individual ones and buy a glass bottle that you use to carry water around in, instead of buying bottles outside. Investing in a thermos and eating leftovers for lunch will save you a packet too.

Shop more - If you can do small shops 2 - 3 times a week, in different shops, you may find you pick up more bargains. Big weekly shopping trips are normally more convenient, but different shops will normally have different things cheaper, so it's worth shopping around. If you shop later in the day, you'll also get the reduced foods, which are still perfectly edible as long as you use them soon.

Bulk Buy – Join with some friends, work out what foods you all like and buy them in bulk at a cash and carry or wholesaler.

Buy more RAW - The more nutritious your food is, the more filling it is, so including raw foods in your diet can provide lasting nourishment which will make you fuller for longer, saving you money on snacks.

Leave the fancy snacks alone - I find that chopped cucumber, cherry tomatoes, oranges, frozen grapes and the occasional corn cake with humus are filling snacks. For others, a slice of cheese, a few nuts, a small cold chicken drumstick or an avocado are ideal and much cheaper than health bars and specialist snacks, that can cost up to £4 for a few mouthfuls, great for an occasional treat, but not everyday if you're on a budget.

DRINK MORE WATER - You may have guessed that I'm quite passionate about this!!! Believe it or not, dehydration can make you feel hungry, so answering hunger pangs with water first can sometimes be the answer, meaning you eat less and save money

Sprout it - This week, if you buy alfalfa seeds, mung beans and chickpeas, then soak them all over night and start sprouting them, by next week you'll have 3 times the quantity of food you started off with, and a highly nutritious feast of sprouts to add to any meal, smoothie or snack. This is one of the cheapest whole food superfoods you can get when you do it yourself. See Step 24 for more details.

Coupon Time – If you have any rewards schemes points, discount vouchers or coupons lying around, now's the time to cash them in. If you have friends that are good at finding coupons and deals, have a chat and see what advice you can pick up.

Step 29 – Work out a food budget you can afford long term and stick to it while eating the best foods, using the tips above for a week

---

To make this step a success, this week I am committed to:

_____

_____

_____

_____

_____

_____

_____

By the end of this week I hope to:

_____

_____

_____

_____

_____

Your Becoming Naturally You Food Steps Action Sheets

Weekly Meal Planner

An easy way to make sure you add healthier wholesome foods to your diet is to make a plan where you include them. This very basic meal planner can be used to plan exactly what you are going to eat for breakfast, lunch or dinner over 5 days, or just to remind you to add certain things to each meal. Have a look at the example given. Copy or reate a table like the one below and complete it.

Day/Meal	Breakfast	Lunch	Dinner
Example	2 glasses of water & lemon 10 mins before breakfast – Lentil soup	Walnut and Mushroom burger with almond mayo	Make half this meal a salad with greens
Day 1			
Day 2			
Day 3			
Day 4			
Day 5			

What Are You Eating

This exercise will help you to see how many real foods vs. processed or non foods you have in your diet. Try to be as honest as you can, this is the only way you'll get a real idea of your current diet – the more non foods you're eating, the more likely it is that you could do with a change. On a piece of paper, create a table like the one below and complete it.

Real Whole Foods - On this side, write the foods you've eaten today that you've made yourself from scratch (i.e not pasta sauce, all purpose seasoning, sauce from a packet, processed, flavoured enhanced etc), you know all the ingredients in them, or they are raw and completely natural	Non Foods - On this side, write the foods you've eaten today that you bought ready made, it came out of a packet, you don't know more than 3 ingredients in it, it's typically described as junk or you know it's a highly processed food, far from its natural state

How do you feel?
Write a few words about how what you've documented above makes you feel (i.e. proud of yourself, surprised, concerned, shocked, embarrassed, ready for a change etc.)

Food and Feelings Diary

This is a simplified but still effective version of the Diet Check Records I use with my clients to find out exactly how the foods they are eating are affecting them.

Just by noting down whether a food made you feel good or bad, then removing foods that constantly make you feel bad and including more of the ones that constantly make you feel good, you can adjust your own diet to make it serve you better.

Have a look at the example for an idea of how to fill it out

Date & Time	What I Ate Or Drank	It made me feel good = √ not good= x	Comments
Wed 8pm	Roast chicken breast, romaine lettuce and sliced tomato & avocado	X	I feel tired and irritable, I'm full but I still desire sweets

Becoming Naturally You

Your Becoming Naturally You Body Steps

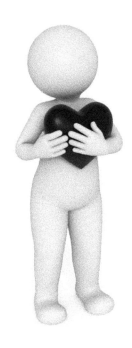

"Don't dwell in illness, create your wellness"
Leah Salmon

Just a quick hit of biology to get you in the mood!!

Your body is made up of billions of cells, which are grouped into tissues, which are grouped into organs, then systems which make up the finished product, you.

As well as having a diet that supports all those billions of cells, there are many things you can do physically that can keep everything working in harmony from a cellular level, because if the cells aren't working properly it will affect the tissues, then organs, then systems, then you get a pain in the behind, sometimes quite literally.

If you are trying to live holistically, it's important to realise that focusing on just one area of your health and well being at any time without supporting the others can make the results you're looking for take longer to show up.

This is precisely why taking a number of steps in many levels of your life over a period of time can prove the most effective way to get real results.

So next we are going to look at 9 steps you can take with your body (plus one bonus step), to support the steps you may have already taken with your mind environment and foods, that will get you to love your Naturally You life.

Step 30 – Get Fit For Success

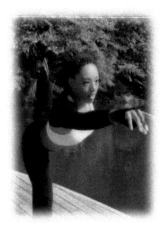

Stretch for success

If you are thinking about getting physical but you've been a bit of a couch potato for a few months, some simple stretches on a daily basis can loosen up your muscles and slowly get you back to match fitness, so when you embark on your training, your body can handle more and recover more easily.

Paul Chek's book 'How to Eat Move and Be Healthy" has an excellent section on stretches that can get you off to a good start.

Hit the ground running by hiring a professional

In the same way there is a diet that works best for your body and it's needs, there's also exercises and stretches that are best for your body. There are a group of highly trained exercises coaches called Chek Exercise Coaches who you can give you a full body assessment before prescribing a personalised exercise plan that suits you to the T!!!

If you're in London visit www.warrenwilliamscoaching.com or visit www.chekconnect.com/app/findpractitioner to find a practitioner in your area worldwide.

If you can't get hold of them, ask around for a recommended fitness coach or personal trainer, preferably one that focuses on functional exercise instead of machine work to help you create a plan and stick to it. African or Kemetic yoga or Crossfit also have well trained trainers you can work with.

Have at least one cool piece of kit
If you need a little motivation to get active, going shopping to get yourself some new trainers, a funky head band or the latest name brand running suit can be just what you need to make your first jog around the park a bit more enjoyable.

Find an exercise you like
It helps if you enjoy the exercise you're going to pursue. If you don't really know what's out there, check out the classes that your local gym has on and try a few out until you find a few you like.

You tube have probably thousands of exercise videos you can try and Pintrest has tons of pins with infographics of exercise routines you can check out. I'd recommend you search for functional, core or gym free body weight exercises on both sites.

Having some variety to your training regime gives you a good chance of working all your muscles.

Do an exercise you don't like
When you don't use a muscle or group of muscles often they become stiff and painful to exercise. So if you find an exercise that works them, it is likely to hurt more than others and this might put you off. But like my osteopath says, "it's likely you don't like it because you really need it". A good exercise coach can give you exercises to work and stretch it safely.

Join a work or local team
If you aren't the sporty type but you are social, why not try and workout socially with your work team or local sports team. Even if

it's just you and a bunch of friends playing basketball or football once a week, or going to a salsa, African or Spanish dance class every Friday night. They are great ways to work out that don't have to involve a leotard, leggings and a head band.

Find the alternative
Without any planning, preparation or change of clothing, you can add little energetic practices to your life.

Use the stairs instead of a lift
Get off the bus one stop early and walk the rest of the way to wherever you are going
Park your car at the other end of the car park, rather than at the door to the supermarket
Wash your own car instead of using a car wash, give it a really good polish and do it all in a time limit so you are forced to work fast but quite hard, no sloppy quick jobs!
Scrub your floors by hand in a time limit
Wash your windows in a time limit
Hoover your house in a time limit
Just for a laugh you could even challenge your children to a race instead of sending them to play outside without you a few times a week.

Step 30 – Do at least 4 of the above this week

Choose a few you know you can easily do and one that might be a bit more challenging. if you have a medical reason not to exercise, seek advice before starting.

To make this step a success, this week I am committed to:

_____

_____

_____

_____

_____

_____

_____

_____

_____

_____

By the end of this week I hope to:

_____

_____

_____

_____

_____

Step 31 – Clean Your Bowels

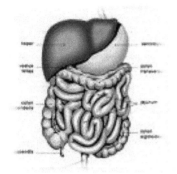

The popular saying 'You are what you eat', has done a great job of increasing people's awareness that everything you eat has an effect on your body and contributes to who you are, your state of health, energy levels, likelihood of developing illnesses, quality of skin, hair, nails and life.

However, what has become very apparent in the health world is that you are what you absorb. Huh isn't that the same thing? If you eat something you absorb it right? Well, not necessarily.

Why do we need to cleanse?

Once you've chewed and swallowed your food and it gets past your stomach and into your bowels, this is where quite a few nutrients in the food are ready to be absorbed into your bloodstream and distributed throughout your body. This is the point at which your food really does its job. But it's also at this point that it can just become another piece of debris that sits on the walls of your bowels waiting to be evacuated.

With all the poor and frequent food combinations, severe lack of water and fibre in our diets and the over consumption of rancid oils, sugar and junk, our bowels, which should be clear and ready to absorb the nutrients from food, are sometimes so heavily clogged with decaying and putrefying waste that got stuck there, that few nutrients can get absorbed. It's like a thick layer of sludge that coats your drains that can eventually block them.

172

When this waste sits in the bowels for long periods of time, it actually gets absorbed into the bloodstream and circulates around the body, resulting in skin eruptions, headaches, tiredness and many more niggling health complaints including a condition called Leaky Gut Syndrome. So regular cleansing is necessary to remove this thick wall of sludge many of us are carrying round.

What are the benefits of cleansing our bowels?
By cleansing your bowels, especially the lower largest part called the colon, you'll absorb more nutrients from your food, remove years of decaying food that could have built up in there and improve your general well being. People have noted feeling more energetic with less cravings and not being constantly hungry. You'll be happy to get on the scales after a cleanse, as you can lose ten's of pounds after a good one.

How can you cleanse your bowels?
After including plenty of water, fresh raw fruit and vegetables to your diet, the two cleansing methods I'd recommend are a lower bowel cleanse using herbs for a week or so to loosen the impacted material and initiate daily stools to be passed, then several enemas over the following week to manually remove the loosened debris.

If you've never done this before, you may benefits from working through this with a natural health coach with experience.

Secondly, you could visit a trained professional Colon hydro therapist. For those who aren't sure, an enema is a small bottle or sometimes a larger bag of warm water or other solution that is connected to a tube that's inserted into your anus and the liquid is passed into your lower colon, to physically clean you out.

This is something you can do at home. Colon hydrotherapy involves gallons of water being pumped into your colon using a special machine, giving a much deeper cleanse that goes higher up into the bowel. This needs to be done by a professional.

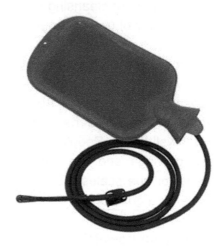

Step 31 – Do an enema or get a colonic

Focus on ensuring your following Steps 13, 15 & 16 for a full 5 days then on the 6th and 7th day, do an enema or get a colonic once on day 6.

There are loads of enema kits to choose from so get one that suits your budget and needs, which will typically come with a full set of instructions. If you book yourself a colonic, at the time of bookings you can ask what's involved and required from you for this.

Either way make sure you take a lactobacillic acidophilus supplement after each one to replace the friendly bacteria you'll wash away.

To make this step a success, this week I am committed to:

_____

_____

_____

_____

_____

_____

_____

_____

_____

_____

_____

By the end of this week I hope to:

_____

_____

_____

_____

_____

Step 32 – Get Your Rest

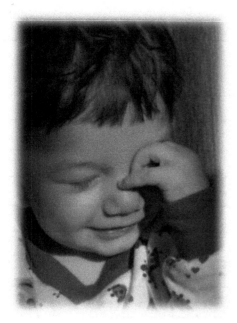

With all the changes you may have already made over the past weeks, your body could probably do with some really restful sleep right now to process all it's experiencing.

A lot of cleansing happens at night so if your sleep is interrupted, so is your body's cleansing and healing time,

When you don't get enough sleep, no matter what you eat, how well you plan or how much water you drink, you are going to eventually feel horrible so here are some tips to help you get some really great 'shut eye'!

Top Tips To Get A Good Night's Sleep

- **Drink some water** about 1hr before you go to sleep. This is better than juice, tea, coffee or hot chocolate as it won't stimulate you in any major way or disrupt your sleep, but it will help add some much needed hydration to your body which is about to enter a night of absorbing nutrients and eliminating waste, both of which benefit from water being present.

- **Turn everything off** – Give your eyes and brain a break from screens and monitors for at least 30mins before you get into bed to make sleep as restful as possible. Unless you're doing something in particular, bedtime isn't the best time to play music or a game on your phone, which can both stimulate rather than relax you. Charging and keeping your devices right next to your bed as you sleep will mean you're absorbing the radiation from them all night so turn them off if possible, even your wifi which fills your home could get turned off. If you can't turn your devices off, keep them as far from your bed as possible.

- **Complete darkness is best**. Invest in some blackout blinds to shield your bedroom from streetlights and if you can't get it completely dark, get an eye mask instead. Studies have showed the darker the room you sleep in, the deeper you sleep.

- **Aim to sleep is from about 10:30pm for about 6-8 hours**. This is the time when most people's organs start the process of assimilating nutrients from the food they've eaten that day, This goes on until about 4am when detoxification processes start, lasting until about 10am, so until 10am or whenever you get hungry, it is best to eat light foods that don't disrupt that detoxification process.

  The smoother this process is, the better your body will function generally, which will of course impact your sleep. Some people will obviously need more or less sleep and the time of year can effect your sleep too, so start with this plan and adjust it to suit you if it's not working. .

- **Control your temperature** - Make sure you are neither too hot nor too cold when you go to sleep. Sleeping with the central heating on or a window wide open can both disrupt your sleep patterns, but a small crack in the window to supply you with fresh air is good.

- **Try not to eat for at least 1 hour before you sleep**. Digesting a heavy or badly combined meal can interfere with your sleep. A green juice or a little protein about 1 hour before you sleep can make your sleep more restful, so find out what works for you, but always wait an hour before sleeping.

- **Lemon or lavender essential oils** can aid a restful and calm sleep, place 1-2 drops on your pillow away from your face before you lie down so you can breathe them in as you drift off.

Step 32 – Get a good night's sleep for a week

Aim to go to bed at 10:30pm and wake up at 6:30am if you can, or just plan it so you get 8hrs sleep a night. If your work time is in the evenings or you normally do housework, pay bills, participate in activities, surf the net or something else during this time, just for a week, find another time to do it.

For more information on the benefits of sleep read "Lights Out" by T.S. Wiley

---

To make this step a success, this week I am committed to:

_____

_____

_____

_____

_____

_____

_____

_____

_____

_____

_____

By the end of this week I hope to:

_____

_____

_____

_____

Step 33 – The Candida Menace

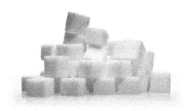 I used to see a nutritionist who worked in a health food shop in London. A lot of my friends went to see her actually as she seemed to know what she was talking about and was quite strict with her advice.

Everyone that went to see her would always leave at least £50 lighter from all the products she recommended, but we did see results. One thing we all realised after a while, was that she had told all of us that we had Candida. We were all recommended the same products and all given the same dietary advice to "kill the Candida", no matter what we presented with.

Once I started training to become a nutritionist, I realised that in fact, virtually everyone has a certain amount of the micro organism Candida in their system. Along with friendly bacteria, they make up the colony of various bacteria in our gut and the rest of our body. Candida actually only become a problem when their numbers become too great and they begin to produce symptoms in our body. Our body sees Candida as a foreign body in large numbers and so when there are too many of them, our immune system begins to fight it off in various ways.

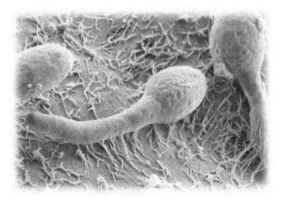

The symptoms produced by Candida overgrowth include, but are by no means limited to:

Fatigue	Drowsiness
Constipation	Diarrhoea
Headaches	Bad breath
Coughing	Wheezing
Joint swelling	Sweet cravings
Irritability	Depression
Nasal congestion	Ringworm
Vaginal itchiness	Nasal discharge
Toenail infections	Vaginal discharge
Fingernail infections	Athletes foot
Frequent/Burning Urination	Dry itchy flaky scalp

As the symptoms are so diverse, it's easy for the overgrowth to be overlooked and just treat the symptoms (i.e take an aspirin for the headaches, get a topical cream for the vaginal itch, chew some gum for the bad breath etc), which leave the root cause untreated.

According to one of my favourite books on this subject 'Candida Albicans' By Leon Chaitow, the 5 main reasons that Candida get out of control are:

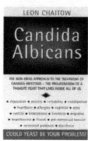

1. Our diet is too rich in simple sugars
2. We have an underlying inherited or acquired deficiency of the immune system
3. It's the long-term effect of exposure to antibiotics in our food (factory farmed animals, or their products such as milk) or that we've taken as medication
4. The aftermath of steroids (hormones) in food (residues found in factory farmed meat and poultry, for example) or as medication (cortisone, 'the pill', etc).
5. Diabetes (many of us are undiagnosed borderline diabetics without even knowing it)

You are also more likely to develop candida or be suffering from it if:
You've had a vaginal birth
You've been on the pill
You've taken antibiotics
You get frequent persistent bacterial infections
You've had fungal infections
You crave bread, sugar & alcohol
You are really bothered by cigarette smoke

The 4 main aspects of any Candida treatment program should be to

1. Reconstitute the friendly bacteria in the bowel – Candida overgrowth simply means that there are too many of them, they are normally kept in check by friendly bacteria, so increasing the friendly bacteria in the bowels will control the Candida overgrowth. Taking lactobacillic acidophilus, a fermented food like sauerkraut or a drink like kefir or kombucha

2. Build your body's immunity – the fact that the Candida were able to become overgrown shows that the immune system was compromised in some way

3. Ensure you have adequate amounts of fibre in your diet – this keeps your bowels clean and well functioning to make Candida over growth less likely

4. Reduce the amount of processed carbs in your diet that are a food source for the candida and suppress the immune system we're working to boost.

Step 33 – Follow the 4 basic steps for a week

Unless you have a swab taken and test it in a lab, the best way to see if you have Candida, is to see if you have the symptoms, then follow the 4 basic steps for 7 days and see if you notice any difference.

As the steps are beneficial to your health anyway, following this step this week is a good idea for everyone.

To make this step a success, this week I am committed to:

_____

_____

_____

_____

_____

_____

_____

_____

_____

By the end of this week I hope to:

_____

_____

_____

_____

_____

Step 34 – Breath Deeply

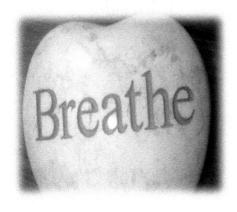

Most people have probably worked out that you need to breathe to live!!! We all know what happens if you were to stop breathing. But did you realise that just because you're breathing enough to keep your heart beating, doesn't mean that you are actually breathing properly?

You breathe in and then breathe out and that's it right? Wrong. It's normally only babies, young children and those that know about energy healing, meditation, martial arts and other holistic practices that are actually breathing properly.

To breathe properly, you need to be inhaling through your nose, filling your abdomen and chest and pushing them out, then breathing out through your mouth while you deflate those areas.

In modern times, being an adult, especially a female, and having a slightly pot belly isn't cool to say the least, but moving your tummy in and out whilst breathing can significantly improve your oxygen intake and is the way we naturally breathed as a child, which is why many babies have little pot bellies. I'm no expert on the complex science of breathing, but the above simple breakdown is based on research from authors such as the great Dr Malachi Z York who's written over 500 hundred books on many subjects, including a book called "The Breath" and "The Mind Scroll" which both talk about the importance of correct breathing.

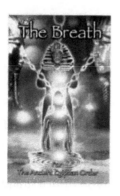
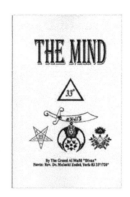

Oxygen is actually a source of energy for our bodies. When we breathe in, the oxygen goes into our lungs then into our blood stream to be carried to all the tissues and organs in the body which use it as an energy source. The process of respiration actually turns oxygen into energy, so when we don't breath properly and take in inadequate amounts of oxygen on a regular basis, we are literally depriving our cells, tissues and organs from one of their energy sources and compromising the amount of energy we could be producing.

When you start any martial arts, meditation or energy healing practice, one of the first things that you'll be taught is how to breathe properly. This is normally so that you can supply all the muscles in the body with the oxygen they need to perform during whatever you'll be practising. Your cells also use oxygen to carry out cleansing of the waste products produced from cellular respiration, another good reason to take in more O2.

It's not only therapeutic to the body, but also very relaxing to just, drop your shoulders, lift your chest, sit up straight and focus on your breathing for a certain amount of time a day

186

Step 34 – Schedule 10 mins 3 times a day during this week to make sure you are breathing deeply

You don't have to stop everything you're doing at these times, when your reminder alarm goes off saying "breathing time", no matter what you're doing (apart from swimming or giving a talk ☺) make sure you are breathing fully & deeply for 10mins.

To make this step a success, this week I am committed to:

_____

_____

_____

_____

_____

_____

By the end of this week I hope to:

_____

_____

_____

_____

Step 35 – Listen To Your Body

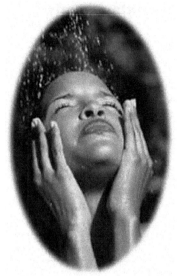

Believe it or not, no aches or pains are natural. So the lump you've had on your chest for the past 10 years that's never given you any problems probably shouldn't be there.

The sharp pain you occasionally get in your side is a sign that something isn't right. That patch of dry skin behind your left knee that flares up during hot weather is something that needs to be checked out.

Many of us have never experienced optimal health and accept the aches and pains we experience as just part of life. Humans are excellent at adapting. So you may have been to the odd retreat or done the occasional 7-day regime that made you feel on top of the world, without any aches, pains, bump or lumps, but as soon as it was over, you fell back into old habits and the old troubles came back too, which you are so used to, you almost expected their return at some point.

This step involves really tuning into your body. Use the table below, pay attention to each of the areas listed to identify ANY aches, pains, dry skin patches, lumps, bumps, growths etc and note down anything that you would consider an unhealthy symptom.

Body Part	Aches / Pains / Stiffness / Weakness / Lumps / Discharges etc
Skin (inc scalp)	*eg. Frequently dry flaky scalp*
Mental	*e.g, Get very easily irritated, complain often*
Neck and spine	*e.g pain in left side of neck when it gets cold*
Chest & Breathing	*e.g. wheeze after eating white bread*
Stomach & lower back	*e.g. constant dull ache on right side of tummy*
Digestion & bowels	*e.g. gas and bloating*
Genitals & Breasts	*e.g. PMS, difficulty holding urine*
Legs and feet	*e.g. athletes foot, dry hard skin under big toe*
Any other	*e.g. always wake up with crusty eyes*

Step 35 – Listen to your body for a week

Use the checklist above to see if any part of your body is trying to tell you something. Do some research to see if you can resolve them or keep them in mind for Step 37.

To make this step a success, this week I am committed to:

_____

_____

_____

_____

_____

_____

_____

_____

By the end of this week I hope to:

_____

_____

Step 36 – Natural Body Care

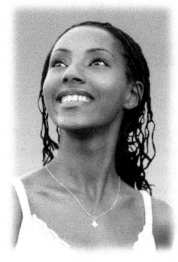

Our skin is the biggest organ in our body. It provides a barrier between the outside world and our internal environment, it can release toxins, water and oils, and it will also absorb things that are put onto it, which is why it is important to know EXACTLY what you put on it.

Just because something is labelled natural, organic, enriching, nourishing, great for skin, doesn't actually make it any of those things. Loose labelling laws and clever marketing has resulted in many of us using products with petrol, dyes, harmful additives and preservatives and even more harmful bleaches and cancer causing chemicals on our bodies and even our children's bodies

Each individual product contains a chemical cocktail, which often only barely passes safety assessment. But when you consider we can use 15 different products every morning, is it any wonder our kidney, liver and skin (3 major detoxification organs) are struggling to keep us toxin free.

If you use soap, toothpaste, mouthwash, dental floss, facial cleanser, toner, moisturiser, shower gel, foundation, lipstick, perfume or aftershave all before leaving the house at 8am and you can't pronounce the ingredients in any of them apart from aqua, there's a problem.

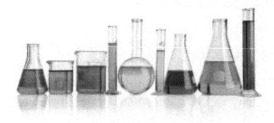

We had beautiful, luscious, supple and gorgeous skin and vibrantly healthy bodies many hundreds of years ago, before the invention of the tons of multi million pound making, synthetic skin care products that fill the supermarket shelves today. We achieved it through proper diet, proper hydration and the use of natural chemical free organic oils, herbs and other earth elements.

If you use a cupboard full of cosmetics currently, or if you get by on a handful of essentials, here are some less harmful, more natural alternative you can add to your skincare range and regime.

Oral Hygiene – Switching to toothpastes and mouthwashes that don't contain fluoride, sugars and artificial flavouring and colouring is a start. But you also have to make sure you prevent oral problems by avoiding eating foods high in refined sugar and things like chewing tobacco. Rinsing your mouth or quickly brushing your teeth after eating highly acidic foods like lemons, oranges and fizzy drinks is another usefu;l step.

At the time of writing I'd recommend Kingfisher fluoride free toothpaste (I love the fennel and the Aloe Vera and Mint) and Fennel Mouthwash by Green People Organic Lifestyle.

Did you know you can make your own mineral rich toothpaste? Check out this simple, natural, harmful chemical free recipe.

Natural Toothpaste Recipe

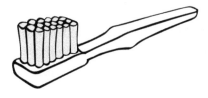

You'll need:
4tbsp of coconut oil
2tbsp of bicarbonate of soda
3 tbsp of xylitol (natural sweetener reported to help gum health)
3 drops of an essential oil like orange, lemon, oregano, tea tree, clove bud, peppermint, cinnamon or grapefruit
2 tbsp of Calcium Carbonate (Optional to make more mineral rich)
2 tbsp of hydrogen peroxide (optional for teeth strengthening and whitening)

Directions
Mix all ingredients together in a bowl, then transfer to a small pot with a lid to keep in the bathroom. Either dip your toothbrush in to pick up a blob or use a wooden lolly stick to put some on your toothbrush at brushing times. As it contains coconut oil, it may harden a bit in cold weather so give it a stir before use if this happens.

I will often make an even simple combination of just coconut oil, bentonite clay, sea salt and bicarbonate of soda in equal portions, which works well too.

Skin Care – Nourishing your skin from the inside out is by far the best way to go. You can do this by simply drinking enough water and making sure you include some essential fatty acids in your diet. Aside from this, very natural and simple moisturisers like pure shea butter, virgin coconut oil and good old olive oil can all do wonders for your skin.

A quick tip for super soft and supple skin is to rub yourself with one of the above oils while your skin is still wet after a warm bath or shower, then gently pat yourself until any excess water comes off

You can make your own body scrub to exfoliate and moisturise your skin by mixing a cup of sea salt with about 1 ½ cups of olive oil and a few drops of whatever essential oil you like (Lavender and Chamomile) for a calming blend or grapefruit or peppermint for a more invigorating blend). Mix everything in a glass jar thoroughly and leave for at least 30 minutes or a few hours preferably before use.

When you finish a bath or shower, take about 2-3 tbsp of the salt scrub and rub it into your skin, avoiding any sensitive areas of course. Rub in a circular movement around the joints and in long sweeping movements on the limbs, up or down in the direction of the heart to stimulate your circulation at the same time. Then rinse it all off under the shower and pat yourself dry.

After a few days of these treatments, you will have skin as soft as a baby's bum and with a glow of sunshine.

Deodorant - I was quite surprised as a teenager to find out the difference between a deodorant and an antiperspirant. A deodorant actually just deodorises the sweat you produce whereas an antiperspirant attempts to stop you sweating altogether by blocking and clogging up the sweat glands with aluminium salts, one of the most toxic heavy metals around. Aluminium has recently been linked to cancer among other things.

I wasn't that clued up as a teenager on anatomy, physiology and health, but that just sounded wrong. I was sure even then that sweating was something we had to do and I was worried about what was going to happen to the sweat if it stayed in my body. My innate fears were well founded. Blocking and clogging the pores with aluminium salts and other chemicals can cause these chemicals to accumulate in the tissue in the underarm and the breast which is close by, which could result in an increased chance of breast cancer.

Several but not all cancer research institutes dispute this claim, but common sense and a number of natural health experts promote that the risk is very real and the natural alternatives are readily available so we don't ever have to put aluminium of all things anywhere near our skin.

There is also the fact that sweating is a natural cooling mechanism and I can never see a reason to interfere that drastically with a natural bodily function unless life is at stake.

I have heard from people that they don't like using deodorants over antiperspirant because half way through the day, they can smell their body odour. This is a sign that they need a cleanse to flush out the toxins in their system, more than a sign that their deodorant isn't effective.

It could simply be that they either didn't wash their underarms properly or even dry them properly before applying the deodorant, so don't be too quick to assume aluminium free deodorants aren't a safe and effective alternative.

Want to try your hand at making your own deodorant? Check out this simple recipe

Natural Chemical Free Deodorant Recipe

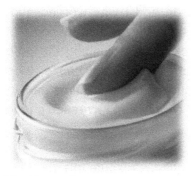

You'll need
3 tbsp of coconut oil
2 tbsp of bentonite clay
1 tbsp of bicarbonate of soda
3 drops of an essential oil for scent (I'd suggest frankincense or cedarwood for men, or rose or geranium for ladies)

Directions
Simply mix all ingredients together well and store in a jar with a lid. After you've washed and dried your armpits well, take a small amount with your fingers and wipe it under your armpits. If you are feeling adventurous, you can get an old deodorant stick container, wash out the inside, wind it to the bottom, pour the mixture into it, then put it in the fridge until it hardens and keep it in the fridge between uses so it stays solid.

Soap – Some of the most dangerous chemicals added to soaps and shampoos are Sodium Lauryl Sulphate (SLS) and Sodium Laureth Sulphate (SLES) and they are found in literally all commercial body washing products. These products are cheap additions to these products that help them to produce lovely bubbles, an important selling feature. Originally, because of their degreasing abilities, these products were used as an industrial factory cleaner.

A study at the Medical College of Georgia, indicated that SLS penetrates into the eyes as well as brain, heart and liver and showed long-term retention in the tissues. The study also indicated that SLS penetrated young children's eyes and prevented them from developing properly and caused cataracts to develop in adults. It may even cause hair loss by attacking the follicles. It's been classified as a drug in bubble baths because it eats away skin protection and causes rashes and infection to occur. It's potentially harmful to skin and hair as it cleans by corrosion and dries skin by stripping the protective lipids from the surface so it can't effectively regulate moisture. But the good news is there are plenty of alternatives

Aside from African black soap (also used as a shampoo), Dudu Osun soap and Castile based soap for skin & hair (i.e. Doctor Bonners Soap), you can do a search for SLS free organic soaps and you'll be spoilt for choice. Based on what you've learnt in this step read a bit about new products you find before purchasing, but if you they are SLS free, organic and unperfumed you should be fine.

Step 36 – Switch to as many natural alternatives to the more harmful body care products as you can for a week

---

197

To make this step a success, this week I am committed to:

_____

_____

_____

_____

_____

_____

_____

_____

_____

_____

By the end of this week I hope to:

_____

_____

_____

_____

_____

Step 37 – Get Yourself Checked

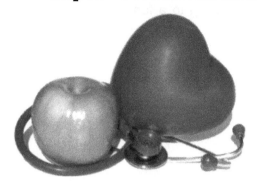

At least twice a year, it's worth giving your body an MOT just to make sure that everything is in tiptop working order.

Normally you'll be able to tell if something isn't working right, but sometimes you won't and finding out a condition in the early stages, before it produces any symptoms can give you a much better chance of effectively treating it with natural methods. Here are some checks you could book yourself in for:

Food Allergy Testing – You can develop food intolerances and allergies at any time and for many reasons, so getting yourself tested at least once is always a good idea. You could be putting your body under unnecessary stress by constantly subjecting it to a food it's intolerant too.

This will over work your body's defences, leading to a general weakening of your system. To date the best food intolerance testing I know of is called Mediator Release Testing or MRT, which can test your sensitivity to up to 150 different foods stuffs. Leap and ELISA testing are also options.

Your local GP is unlikely to give you an allergy test unless they are confident you definitely have an intolerance and many doctors don't give much regard for the power of food and diet changes, so you're more than likely going to have to get it done privately.

You can also perform a quick self-test on yourself or children to see if the body is in someway reacting to a food by simply using your pulse.

Food Sensitivity Pulse Testing

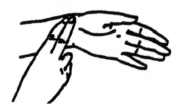

Directions
1. Either perform this test first thing in the morning before you've eaten anything or 2hrs after eating.
2. Wash your mouth out with plain water
3. Get the food you want to test ready near you with a Testing Chart (see below), a pen (that works!!!) and a clock
4. Take your pulse at your wrist by placing your index and middle fingers either side of the veins in the middle of the inside of your wrist where your wrist dips down. Press down until you can feel your pulse, don't use your thumb to check your pulse as it has it's own pulse which may confuse you. Once you've found your pulse, count how many times it pulses over a full minute and records the result in the "Pre test" column next to the food your testing
5. Now take the food you want to test and put it in your mouth for a full minute so you get a good taste of it. There's no need to swallow it though.
6. After the minute, remove the food from your mouth and take your pulse again for a full minute. If it goes up or down by more than 5 beats a minute, your body is reacting to it in some way.

It's best to test just one food at a time, so instead of taking a bite of chicken sandwich, test the bread, chicken, mayo and lettuce all separately. This is because if you react, you won't know which ingredient gave you the reaction. You'll have to wait a couple of hours before testing another food so it's best to test them on different days or one in the morning and another in the evening.

Getting a reaction of more than 5 beats a minute doesn't mean the food is fatally dangerous to eat, but I'd advise removing it from your diet for at least 3 weeks to see if any symptoms improve and check if any big reactions happen when you reintroduce it. You may also want to retest yourself periodically to see if anything changes. Use the table below to record your results (or you can make a copy of the page or make a similar table to use)

Pulse Testing Results Table

Date & Time	Food/Drink	Pre Test Pulse	Post Test Pulse	Difference in Pulse

Hair Mineral Analysis – Even if you live in the heart of the countryside, surrounded by rolling green hills, natural spring waters and organic crops, in these days and times the likelihood is that you have been exposed to the toxic heavy metals that are found in the water, food and air all around us. Once these accumulate in our body, they can disrupt our mineral absorption, immune system and general well being. A Hair Mineral Test can reveal mineral deficiencies and the levels of heavy metals in your system, so you can boost any deficiencies and detox heavy metals that appear in high levels.

Metabolic Typing Retest - If you've read this far into the book and you still haven't found out your metabolic type (refer to Step 23), what are you waiting for?!? As you're likely to change from your functioning metabolic type to your genetic metabolic type at some point, it's best to get yourself retested at least twice a year. This way you'll be able to adapt your diet to meet your body's most current nutritional needs and always thrive on your food. Your fuctional MT is the type your body is when first tested that's based on your current environment, stress levels, illnesses, energy levels etc and your genetic MT is the way you function genetically.

Energy Healer – Have you ever had an energy healer do work on your energetic body, which some refer to as an aura, auric field or spiritual body? Using practices like Reiki, Reiju, Sekhem and Cartouche mastery, energy healers can realign, open up and re-energise your chakras which can become shut down or closed for various reasons. We spend a lot of time on our physical bodies; time should also be spent ensuring our spiritual bodies are in good working order. For safety, I'd advise you work with someone who's been recommended to you.

Corrective Exercise Coach – Anyone can do a 6 week exercise coaching course and put an exercise plan together for you with little or no real experience to back up their paperwork, but if you really want to know what's going on with your muscles, posture, joints and skeleton, go back to Step 30 where I talk more about CHEK certified exercise coaches. They will be able to assess you thoroughly, put together an exercise plan for you that will correct imbalances naturally, hence the term corrective exercise. In my opinion, these guys are top class in this field.

Holistic Dentists, Opticians & Doctors – You can find quite a few holistic mercury free dentists to give your teeth and gums a check twice a year and an optician can pick up on any problems with your eyes before they develop, which you can use herbs, bates method exercises or maybe even pinhole glasses to rectify.

Whilst I don't agree with most of the treatments doctors propose for diseases they find, they can help you detect conditions in their early stages, which you can then treat using natural methods. If you are lucky enough to find a holistically minded doctor and optician, they can even steer you in the right direction to treat it holistically too.

Step 37 – Decide 3 ways to check yourself this week

If you choose 3 specialists, aim to see one of them each month for the next 3 months. If the price of the appointments is an issue, firstly, you'll normally pay on the day, so you'll have time to save for them as you're just booking them now. Secondly, special offers to see complementary therapists pop up on Groupon type sites all the time. Some are also more affordable they you may think. .

To make this step a success, this week I am committed to:

_____

_____

_____

_____

_____

_____

_____

_____

_____

_____

_____

By the end of this week I hope to:

_____

_____

_____

_____

_____

Step 38 – Everybody Loves The Sunshine

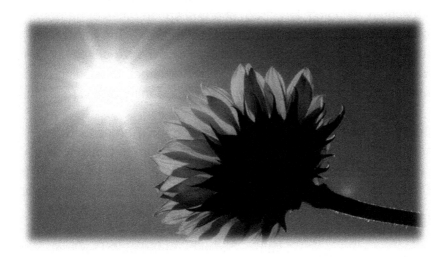

With so many great things to do inside, many of us only leave the house to do the shopping (if we don't use internet shopping), go to work (before we get into our car, bus or train) or put the bin out on Wednesday evening (Oh, I knew I forgot something, oh well there's always next week!).

There's television, computer games, the internet and high tech entertainment systems all enticing you to stay in, well now it's time to go outside WITHOUT looking at your smartphone while you're out there.

Do you remember the episode of The Simpsons when one of the children's favourite cartoons was changed and the children didn't like it anymore? You saw them all wonder what to do now there was nothing good on TV, then emerge from their homes rubbing their eyes to adjust to the sunlight and rediscover the great outdoors again.

Encourage your children to spend time outside daily, using their imagination to create games or just enjoying the old classics like, hopscotch, skipping, leap frog, egg and spoon races or garden toys to play and explore, while they get to take in the rays of the sun. Encourage yourself to be outside with them if possible or find ways to do more outside in the sunlight, whether it's reading, walking, running, walking to the shops, gardening or just relaxing.

Being exposed to the rays of the sun is actually prescribed by natural health practitioners. Adequate exposure to sunlight on a daily basis is reported to decrease the risk of cancer by up to 70%, it helps your body to naturally produce vitamin D, which keeps your bones and teeth strong whilst supporting your immune system.

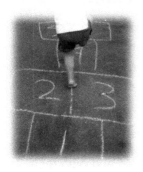

Vitamin D is very important for optimal health. Dietary sources of Vitamin D include mackerel, salmon, sardines, cod liver oil and egg yolks, but exposing just 20% of your body to sunlight, not necessarily hot sunny weather, just the light from the sun, for 15 - 20 minutes a day is enough to provide you with all the vitamin D you need.

Longer periods of time are needed if you are melanin dominant with darker skin. Your melanin can filter the dangerous UV rays from the sun, which allows you to spend much longer in the sun anyway. Deficiencies in vitamin D can lead to depression, Seasonal Affective Disorder (SAD) and increased risk of cancer, allergies, obesity and skin conditions.

You can't get the same affect by being indoors and having the curtains open as the glass blocks the direct contact of your skin to the rays, you actually need to get out and bathe in it.

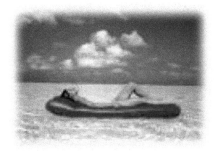

If you are in a relatively unpolluted area, you can use your time outside to enjoy breathing in some fresh air, again many of us are inside breathing in air conditioned air which can carry around everyone's bugs and bacteria's, or stagnant air if you are in a sealed room.

Step 38 – Make sure you get out into the sunlight for at least 1 hour in total a day for a week

---

If you get to this step in summer, lucky you!!! If you're reading this in the midst of a very cold winter, not so lucky.

Do your best and break the hours up into 4x 15min intervals if it makes it better. A brisk walk somewhere, making your phone calls outside or just being at an open window (be very safe) while it's open will do. Just let the sunlight touch your skin.

To make this step a success, this week I am committed to:

_____

_____

_____

_____

_____

_____

_____

_____

_____

_____

By the end of this week I hope to:

_____

_____

_____

_____

_____

Step 39 – So Now What?

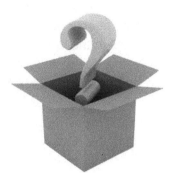

We're finally here, your 39th week!!!! I'm hoping during this time you've implemented changes, liked some, absolutely loved others, felt many improvements in your mind body and spirit and learned much about your body while Becoming Naturally You.

But now what? What should you do with all the energy you have, all the knowledge you've acquired, all the freedom you've found.

There are coaches who devote whole talks and seminars to this one subject because it is so expansive, but here are some things to consider.

1. Don't stop now

Now that you've experienced what being Naturally You is, and what feeling healthier and more vibrant can feel like, don't let it become just another thing you've tried and stopped. Aim to implement as many of these steps into your life on a more permanent basis as you can. If you have benefited from following them for a week or 2, imagine how you'd feel if you lived them. Well, don't just wonder, do it.

You can do this by using the plans at the end of this book. Once you've finished one, start another so it becomes a cycle of working on one or two things a week constantly until they stick.

2. Channel It

If you don't harness or channel the new found energy you've obtained by following these steps, it can become overwhelming to your system and to just feel normal again, people will use food, drugs or behaviours to suppress and stuff down the vibrant energy they have. Please don't do this, if you've tried even half of these points and felt benefits, it would be such a shame to go back now.

Continue the process of Becoming Naturally You by deciding what area of your life to nourish and fulfil now. Maybe now you can get that new job, find the perfect partner, start a family or whatever you feel is the next area that needs attention, let this energy fuel your next phase of personal, mental and professional development.

3. Share the good news

If you've enjoyed this experience and know others that could benefit from it, spread the good news, you can become the inspiration someone else needs to improve their lives.

You don't need to become the next Gillian Michaels or Anthony Robbins, but one of the best things you can do is spread good news (the news channels do a good enough job at spreading bad news, it's time to even the score), put a smile on someone's face and a spring in their step, encourage them that because you were able to do it, there's no reason they can't do it too.

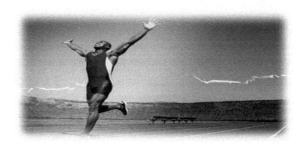

4. Praise your achievements and plan more

At this stage in the game, take a moment to look back on what you've achieved in the 3 areas you've been working on and then

The improvements I've made in my mind and thoughts since the beginning of this program are:

_____

_____

_____

The other improvements I'd like to work on in my mind and thoughts are

_____

_____

_____

The improvements I've made in my environment since the beginning of this program are:

_____

_____

_____

The other improvements I'd like to work on in my environment are:

_____

_____

_____

Becoming Naturally You

The improvements I've made with my food since the beginning of this program are:

_____

_____

_____

The other improvements I'd like to work on with my foods are:

_____

_____

_____

The improvements I've made in my body since the beginning of this program are:

_____

_____

_____

The other improvements I'd like to work on in my body are:

_____

_____

_____

Step 39 – Work out where go from here this week to continue the process of Becoming Naturally You

Spend this week deciding where you can go from here, personally, professionally, mentally and spiritually, even if that means starting the whole 39 weeks again using a different plan

To make this step a success, this week I am committed to:

_____

_____

_____

_____

_____

_____

By the end of this week I hope to:

_____

_____

_____

Your Becoming Naturally You Body Steps Action Sheets

What Can Your Body Do

This little exercise gives you a quick fun look at what your body can actually do. Whether you think you're healthy and agile or unhealthy and stiff, you might think differently in the next 10 minutes. Please don't do anything you're not comfortable with, I don't want you to finish reading this book from a stretcher. Just enjoy for now and test yourself again in the next 3 months to see if there's been any improvement

Can you ...?	Now Yes / No	In 3mths Yes / No
1. Touch your toes?		
2. Look down and see your toes without bending over your tummy?		
3. Do the splits in either direction?		
4. Rotate your head around slowly, with full range of motion and feel no pain?		
5. Stand on one leg without failing over for 10 seconds?		
6. Walk up a flight of stairs without getting out of breath?		

7. Run up a flight of stairs without getting out of breath?		
8. Do 10 sit ups?		
9. Do 10 press ups?		
10. Spin around on the spot without getting dizzy?		
11. Spin a hula hoop around your waist?		
12. Win a race with a 10 year old or someone 10yrs younger than you?		
13. 10 start jumps		
14. Hold your own body weight by hanging from something like a bar, children's swing (make sure it's something that can definitely hold your weight without breaking)		
15. Do a hand stand		
16. Do a crab		
17. Do a cartwheel		

Body Vision Board

If you go back to Step 10, we looked at what a vision board is and the benefits of using one.

Remember they are a great way to motivate and inspire change and growth in you. Here's I'm going to ask you to make a simple one just based on your body and we'll be using words instead of pictures to create the vision.

In this exercise, you have 2 outlines of a body below to work on. On the body to the left (Me Now) write words that you feel describe your body parts now, then on the body on the right (3mths later, look at me now!!!), write words to describe how you want that same body part to look, feel or be by then.

When I did this exercise, along the upper arm on the Me Now body I wrote 'soft and wobbly' and then on the 3mths later body on the same part I wrote firm and muscular.

A client once wrote "Peppa pig" next to her leg on the Me Now body and "Jennifer Lopez" on the 3mths later body!!! A memorable description that puts a smile on your face is always a winner.

So now it's your go!!!

Me Now

3mths later, look at me now!!!

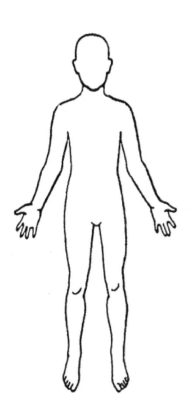
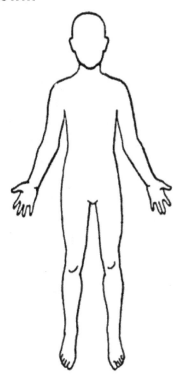

Write a few words describing how you feel about what you've written on each body:

The Becoming Naturally You Plans

Now we come to the good part, actually working out how you're going to implement the information you've read so far. In the next few pages I have set out 4 possible ways you can follow the plan. Choose the one you want to follow, print it out and stick it up everywhere so you can easily keep on track. For the techies among us, you can even schedule each step into the calendar on your computer, smart phone or tablet, with a reminder alarm at the beginning of each week to make it super easy for you to remember and implement each step. The plans on the following pages are:

Plan 1 – The Cover to Cover Plan
This plan follows the steps as they are set out in the book. The benefit of this plan is you get to focus on one area at a time, which some will find easier.

Plan 2 – The Fast Track Plan
This plan is the same as above, but you do 2 steps per week, finish in 20 instead of 39 weeks and see result quicker, but you obviously have more to focus on each week. It's more challenging, but also more rewarding and very manageable if you're up for it.

Plan 3 – The Variety Plan
This plan mixes all the points up, a bit like this: The benefit of this plan is that you get to work on different areas each week, which might make it a bit more interesting for you

Plan 4 – My 39 Steps Plan
This plan has been left blank so that you can decide the order of the steps. If you already know what you want to work on first, this is the best one for you.

Plan 1 - The Cover to Cover Plan

Week	Step	Done	How did it go
1	Potential Trouble Source		
2	Write From The Heart		
3	Stress Busting		
4	Healthy Home Makeover		
5	Affirmations		
6	Do What You Love		
7	The Real Enemy		
8	Social & Supported		
9	Colour Therapy		
10	Vision Board Your Goals		
11	Bribery & Corruption		
12	The 3 Nasties		
13	Wonderful Water		
14	Get Those Juices Flowing		
15	There Are No Teeth in Your Tummy		
16	A Whole Lot Better		
17	Get It Fresh & Local		
18	Know Your Seasons		
19	Mix It Up A Bit		
20	Rawsome		
21	Get Your Greens		
22	Get It Organic		
23	Eat Right For Your Body Type		
24	Sprout It		
25	Herbs, Spices & Salts		
26	Know Your Oils		
27	Be Snack Savvy		
28	Fail To Plan, Plan To Fail		
29	Know How To Work A Budget		
30	Get Fit For Success		
31	Clean Your Bowels		
32	Get Your Rest		

Becoming Naturally You

33	The Candida Menace		
34	Breathe Deeply		
35	Listen To Your Body		
36	Natural Body Care		
37	Get Yourself Checked		
38	Everybody Loves The Sunshine		
39	So Now What?		

39 weeks later....
Write a bit about how you feel after working through all the steps to Becoming Naturally You

Plan 2 - The Fast Track Plan

Week	Small Step	Done	How did it go
1	Potential Trouble Source Write From The Heart		
2	Stress Busting Healthy Home Makeover		
3	Affirmations Do What You Love		
4	The Real Enemy Social & Supported		
5	Colour Therapy Vision Board Your Goals		
6	Bribery & Corruption The 3 Nasties		
7	Wonderful Water Get Those Juices Flowing		
8	There Are No Teeth in Your Tummy A Whole Lot Better		
9	Get It Fresh & Local Know Your Seasons		
10	Mix It Up A Bit Rawsome		
11	Get Your Greens Get It Organic		
12	Eat Right For Your Body Type Sprout It		
13	Herbs, Spices & Salts Know Your Oils		
14	Be Snack Savvy Fail To Plan, Plan To Fail		
15	Know How To Work A Budget Get Fit For Success		
16	Clean Your Bowels Get Your Rest		

17	The Candida Menace Breathe Deeply		
18	Listen To Your Body Natural Body Care		
19	Get Yourself Checked Everybody Loves The Sunshine		
20	So Now What?		

20 weeks later....

Write a bit about how you feel after working through all the steps to Becoming Naturally You

Plan 3 - The Variety Plan

Week	Small Step	Done	How did it go
1	Potential Trouble Sources		
2	The 3 Nasties		
3	Wonderful Water		
4	Get Fit For Success		
5	Journaling		
6	Stress Busting		
7	Get Your Juices Flowing		
8	There's No Teeth In Your Tummy		
9	Clean Your Colon		
10	Healthy Home Makeover		
11	A Whole Lot Better		
12	Get It Fresh & Local		
13	Get Your Rest		
14	Affirmations		
15	Do What You Love		
16	Know Your Seasons		
17	Mix It Up		
18	The Candida Menace		
19	The Real Enemy		
20	Rawsome		
21	Get Your Greens		
22	Breathe Deeply		
23	Social & Supported		
24	Get It Organic		
25	Eat Right For Your Body Type		
26	Listen To Your Body		
27	Colour Therapy		
28	Sprout It		
29	Herbs, Spices & Salts		
30	Natural Body Care		
31	Know Your Goals With A Vision Board		
32	Know Your Oils		

33	Be Snack Savvy		
34	Get Yourself Checked		
35	Bribery & Corruption		
36	Fail To Plan, Plan To Fail		
37	Know How To Work A Budget		
38	Everybody Loves The Sunshine		
39	So Now What?		

39 weeks later....
Write a bit about how you feel after working through all the steps to
Becoming Naturally You

Plan 4 - My 39 Steps Plan

Week	Small Step	Done	How did it go
1			
2			
3			
4			
5			
6			
7			
8			
9			
10			
11			
12			
13			
14			
15			
16			
17			

18			
19			
20			
21			
22			
23			
24			
25			
26			
27			
28			
29			
30			
31			
32			
33			
34			
35			

Becoming Naturally You

36			
37			
38			
39			

39 weeks later....
Write a bit about how you feel after working through all the steps
to Becoming Naturally You

On a final note......

I sincerely hope you have enjoyed reading this as much as I have enjoyed putting it together.

I hope it benefits your life and encourages you to make steps towards better mental, physical, emotional and spiritual health so you can start loving life and Becoming Naturally You.

Before first releasing this book, I had been planning to release it for years, but for one reason or the other it didn't happen. In retrospect, I have realised that everything I plan to do, manifests just when it should and not a moment before.

If you find your life follows this pattern too, maybe you are reading this at the precise time that your universe will support any decision you make, that will promote your growth.

I made a decision a few years ago that I wanted to do as much as I could to share my knowledge with the world, so that everyone I touch can experience what it is to be truly happy with themselves and their life, nourished and fulfilled on every level, even for a short time. I know that by making steps towards living a healthier lifestyle, you can experience true happiness and contentment and Become Naturally You.

If you take one thing from this book, let it be that small changes on a regular basis can yield great results, don't ever feel that a better life is out of your reach because it's too much hard work, costs too much or will take too long to feel the difference.

None of this could be further from the truth. The steps in this book are easy to implement, many of them require an investment of time and not money and you'll feel the differences in a number of weeks if not days.

If you start any of the plans and stop before you get through all the points, for any reason, don't worry about it. When you feel you're ready again, start again, maybe on a different plan this time, maybe without using any of the plans at all.

Start each week by randomly picking a number from 1 – 39 and do that step. There's no pressure, no wrong or right way to do this. It's all about you, finding the way that is comfortable for you, to love your life.

Thank you for taking this journey with me.

Take care and stay healthy.

Leah

Leah Salmon
The Naturally You Coach

Bibliography

The Mind *By Dr Malachi Z York*
Candida Albicans *By Leon Chaitow*
Super Juice *By Michael Van Straten*
Fats That Heal, Fats That Kill *By Udo Erasmus*
The Metabolic Typing Diet *By William Wolcott*
How To Eat Move and Be Healthy *By Paul Chek*
Your Bodies Many Cries For Water *By Dr Batmanghelidj*
How To Get Started On Raw Foods *By Karen Knowler*
Your Potential *By Dr Malachi Z York*
Entrepreneur to Ultrapreneur Julian Hall
Budget Behaviour Belief – Leah Salmon

Recommended Websites For Natural Health, Personal Development & Starting Your Own Business

TheNaturallyYouCoach.com
AmunUniversity.com
Undergroudwellness.com
Wellnessmama.com
Balancedbites.com
TonyGaskins.com
MotivatingTheMasses.com
MarieForleo.com
Julianhall.com

About the Author
Leah Salmon – The Naturally You Coach

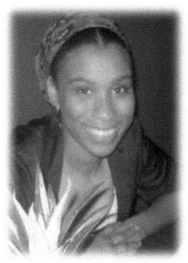

Leah is a passionate motivational and informative speaker, coach, bestselling author of 6 books, founder of The Naturally You Day, raw food workshop facilitator and natural health enthusiast, Leah has worked with people of all ages worldwide over the past 11 years, helping them to use their foods, natural remedies, lifestyle changes and their mindset to boost their health.

More recently, Leah began to focus on helping busy parents professionals and business owners like herself to find time and motivation to achieve their health and life goals and to become nourished and fulfilled on every level or what she calls Becoming Naturally You.

Her journey into natural health and nutrition began when she was just 11 years old when she decided to become vegetarian. Her stressful, soya and junk food filled teens resulted in her developing a concerning gynaecological condition.

After seeking help from doctors who dismissed her condition, she began studying nutrition, aromatherapy and herbal medicine and managed to cure herself using herbs and foods. This sparked her passion to help others use the power of nature and coaching, as she had done, to free themselves of illness, so they didn't need to suffer as she had done.

The biggest message that Leah wants to spread is that improving your health naturally, using whole natural foods is much easier that many people think, you don't have to put up with your health conditions or be bound to a life on medication to manage symptoms.

Vibrant health is not found in a pill, surgery, harmful chemical or crash fad diet, but in living a life that's Naturally You. You can break free from disease, live a fulfilling and rich life and achieve your health goals and most importantly, with support, there's nothing you can't achieve.

Leah runs private & group coaching programs, has an active YouTube channel, a popular free ezine, home study courses and currently has 6 books 5 of which have hit the Amazon best seller list and more coming soon to her site www.TheNaturallyYouCoach.com

To connect with and find out more about Leah, go to:

www.thenaturallyyoucoach.com
leah@thenaturallyyoucoach.com

You can also find her on
Facebook – www.facebook.com/leahthenaturallyyoucoach
www.Facebook.com/groups/melanatedamazingwomen
Pintrest – www.pintrest.com/naturalyoucoach
Twitter – www.twitter.com/naturalyoucoach
You Tube - www.youtube.com/user/NaturallyYouCoach
Instagram - @naturallyyoucoach

More books from TheNaturallyYouCoach.com/shop

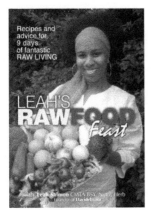

"Leah's Raw Food Feast" Over 100 delicious recipes, tips, advice and plans to help you eat more healthy raw food.

All recipes are free from gluten, wheat, dairy, processed sugar, fish, poultry & meat, but full of flavor and nutrients.

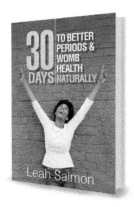

"30 Days To Better Periods & Womb Health"
A simple thorough guide to using foods, herbs, oils, lifestyle changes and other natural practices to experience better periods and womb health in just 30 days.

Lightning Source UK Ltd.
Milton Keynes UK
UKHW020647051218
333453UK00003B/118/P